Working methods in neuropsychopharmacology

Studies in neuroscience

Series editor Dr. William Winlow, *Dept. of Physiology, University of Leeds, LS2 9NQ,* UK

Neuroscience is one of the major growth areas in the biological sciences and draws both techniques and ideas from many other scientific disciplines. The eclectic nature of neuroscience has given it great intellectual appeal, but has slowed its development as a discipline in its own right. *Studies in neuroscience* will present both monographs and multiauthor volumes drawn from the whole range of the subject and will bring together the subdisciplines that have arisen from the recent explosive development of the neurosciences.

Studies in neuroscience will include contributors from molecular and cellular neurobiology, developmental neuroscience (including tissue culture), neural networks and systems research (both clinical and basic) and behavioural neuroscience (including ethology). The series is designed to appeal to research workers in clinical and basic neuroscience, their graduate students and advanced undergraduates with an interest in the subject.

The neurobiology of pain
ed. A.V. Holden *and* W. Winlow

The neurobiology of dopamine systems
ed. W. Winlow *and* Markstein

Other volumes are in preparation

Working methods in neuropsychopharmacology

A team approach

Edited by   M.H. Joseph *and* J.L. Waddington

Manchester University Press

Published by
Manchester University Press
Oxford Road, Manchester M13 9PL, UK

British Library cataloguing in publication data
Working methods in neuropsychopharmacology:
 a team approach. — (Studies in neuroscience)
 1. Psychopharmacology
 I. Joseph, M.H.   I. Waddington, J.L.
 III. Series
 615'.78   RC483

ISBN 0 7190 2245 2 *hardback*

Typeset in Hong Kong by Graphicraft Typesetter Ltd

Printed and bound in Great Britain by
Biddles Ltd, Guildford and King's Lynn

Contents

Preface

An important area of applied psychopharmacology is the study of the drugs used in the treatment of neuropsychiatric disorders, their effects on the transmitter systems of the brain, and the normal and abnormal function of those brain systems in animals and in humans. This calls for the use of techniques derived from disciplines which were initially separate: biochemistry, physiology, anatomy, psychiatry, neurology, ethology, as well as from pharmacology and psychology. Individual investigators, particularly at the postgraduate and post-doctoral level, may need to learn techniques quite different to those covered during their own training. Even where they are fortunate enough to work in multidisciplinary groups, each member of the team often needs to acquire some understanding of the rationale behind the methods used by the others.

The contributors to this book are drawn from past and present members of the Division of Psychiatry at the Medical Research Council's Clinical Research Centre in Harrow. This is a multidisciplinary research unit that has contributed to the development of a wide range of techniques over the past several years, and used them to address problems in psychopharmacology and biological psychiatry. The qualifications of each of the authors are drawn from one or more of the disciplines mentioned above. Our experience in our own research, and in supervising that of others, made us feel the need for a book which described basic techniques in this area for investigators originally trained in various different disciplines.

While reviews of methods are frequently written they are usually aimed primarily at those already working in the same discipline, who use a common vocabulary (even if they sometimes cannot agree on a dictionary) and common preconceptions. In many reviews the available space is used to give a comprehensive survey, rather than detailed procedures for particular methods. Individual research papers, on the other hand, give considerable details about a particular method but may lack contextual information; *why* such and such was done, and whether alternative approaches were considered. Also they usually describe the situation where all the apparatus is installed and working well, rather than how problems were solved to bring about that desirable situation.

The aims of the present work are therefore to complement available publications by providing practical information useful to those wishing to use, or become familiar with, a variety of particular, widely used methods in one area of psychopharmacology. Each chapter is not designed to be a comprehensive review of available methods; rather it contains introductory material to set the method in context, both for the specialist and the non-specialist in that field, and a detailed practical description of how particular techniques are performed. Jargon words are avoided, or explained as appropriate. The implication is not that this is the only way to do it, but that the method described is up-to-date, practicable and has been in regular use by the authors of that chapter. Hence our title: working methods. Where appropriate, the chapters also include sections on trouble-shooting; the priceless information about what is most likely to go wrong, and how to deal with it, that is usually omitted in a 'scientific' paper. The aim here has been to provide something of the benefit of discussing practical problems with someone who has the technique up and running.

The first three chapters illustrate the increasing complexity of behavioural assessment procedures as one progresses phylogenetically from rodents, through primates, to humans as subjects for psychopharmacological research. At each level there are particular experimental problems, the nature of which change with the characteristics of the species under investigation and with the range and subtlety of the observable behaviour. Throughout these first three chapters there is a common emphasis on procedures for the assessment of motor behaviour, to provide a consistent theme on which to base these comparisons.

The fourth chapter concerns itself with procedures for the sampling of tissue and body fluids, usually for neurochemical assays and often subsequent to behavioural studies. Based on the arrangement of the first three chapters, techniques for obtaining such material from both animal and human subjects are described. Possible legal and ethical implications and restrictions are also indicated, as being of special concern to those working with primate or human subjects.

The fifth and sixth chapters cover neurochemical techniques that are commonly applied to such samples. Again, the techniques are presented in a manner which is applicable to samples obtained from either animal or human subjects. In addition to the actual procedures themselves, the authors present accounts of the difficulties they have encountered in applying them to the various materials, and the means adopted to overcome them. Often, neurochemical studies will be natural counterparts to behavioural investigations. One of the most powerful approaches in psychopharmacology is such a combination in systematically designed studies. This again reflects the multidisciplinary concept advocated above, and re-emphasises the need for the scientist to acquire expertise in areas distinct from his or her own training.

The final chapter covers a topic that is not commonly treated in this context but which we feel makes an important contribution to the outcome of psychopharmacological research. Keeping track of the data one has painstakingly collected can be a major problem, especially in large multi-disciplinary studies with inputs from, for example, psychiatrists, pharmacologists and biochemists. Modern techniques can greatly aid the acquisition, storage, retrieval and preliminary evaluation of large amounts of data, before they are exposed to the rigours of statistical analysis.

We intend this volume to be suitable for use both in the laboratory and in the clinic, as well as for consultation in the library or office. It is intended not only to offer guidance to those entering new areas of psychopharmacology, but also to help their appreciation of the problems encountered by their colleagues in related and perhaps ultimately collaborative ventures. We hope it might encourage such associations.

We must record our thanks to the Medical Research Council and particularly to Dr T. J. Crow, Head of the Division of Psychiatry at the Clinical Research Centre, for providing us with the opportunity to work in this closely collaborating team drawn from different disciplines. Dr Crow also provided us with the initial impetus to organise this book.

Michael Joseph
John Waddington

Foreword

It is arguable that with the possible exception of molecular genetics no biological discipline has had greater success in the past 30 years than psychopharmacology; even in this comparison its practical achievements in therapy (the introduction of antipsychotic drugs, antidepressants and lithium) have probably been more substantial. Its success is reflected in a burgeoning literature and a rapid increase in the number of scientists who consider themselves as in some sense psychopharmacologists. Yet it is *par excellence* a collaborative discipline created by the coming together of workers of diverse backgrounds in neurochemistry and psychology, in computing techniques and neuroanatomy, and in clinical psychiatry as well as pharmacology itself. Only in so far as workers in these disciplines have been able to understand and acquire techniques from, or at least to co-operate with workers in, scientific traditions other than their own, does psychopharmacology exist.

The success of the discipline is closely linked to the rise of the neurohumoural hypothesis — the concept that neurones intercommunicate by chemical messengers and that the actions of drugs upon the nervous system can be understood in terms of their abilities to influence mechanisms of synthesis and release of transmitters and their actions upon specific receptor substances. The complexity of the chemical topography of transmitter systems is being revealed by mapping studies, and these provide a framework for a selective anatomical approach to the pharmacology of the nervous system. For this reason pharmacologists and neurochemists have become excited and informed about neuroanatomy in a way which seemed inconceivable ten years ago. Stereotaxic lesioning and injection techniques based upon histochemical mapping studies have become types of expertise in high demand; the potential and limitations of these methods have not yet been reached. At the same time interest is increasing in studies of the nervous system at a gross functional level. Whereas much basic electrophysiological work on single neurones continues, there is a need to understand the results on a larger scale in terms of an interaction between anatomical systems and the role of these systems in the function of the nervous system as a whole. It is for this reason that psychology as the scientific study of behaviour has enjoyed a renaissance at least as far as it can be applied to the analysis of changes resulting from experimental interventions in brain systems. Experimental neuropsychology is well established; neurochemical psychology is in its infancy.

It is a curious fact that major advances in treatment (e.g. the introduction of neuroleptic drugs and lithium) have occurred on an entirely empirical basis. Serendipitous clinical observations have led to the introduction of treatments which are surprisingly effective, and whose efficacy requires explanation. Much of the drive behind current psychopharmacological research arises from a desire to find adequate explanations for the efficacy of current treatments, to determine what light this may throw on the nature of the disease processes in major mental disorders, and to improve on these treatments. In this way has arisen an interaction between clinical and experimental approaches to the problems of psychiatric disease. A logical development is the application of laboratory techniques to the study of the disease itself, principally by the chemical study of body fluids (e.g. urine, blood and cerebrospinal fluid) and postmortem brain tissue from patients with disease. The practical difficulties of the crucial step from the basic laboratory hypothesis to the patient with the disease are often exaggerated, and the hypothesis remains untested. Except that some observation is made on material from a patient with the disease, or a prediction is made concerning his response to a particular pharmacological agent, the notion that the disease is being investigated remains insubstantial. Animal models take us far but failure to test the predictions they generate in the case to which they are intended to apply perpetuates error. No psychopharmacologist can afford to be without the clinical contacts with whose collaboration he may be able to eliminate the hypotheses that retard progress in the field as a whole.

Some revolutions in techniques have dramatically extended the range of research and made it much more practicable. Two such advances are ligand binding assays and high-performance liquid chromatography. The former have opened up the field of receptor research and have made possible a range of studies on brain tissue on questions that previously appeared entirely speculative; the latter has made easier, more precise and much more efficient the detection of substances whose assay was previously a highly technical and recondite pursuit. The benefits of the application of computers to data processing are perhaps too obvious and widely appreciated to require comment but the problems of preparation and organisation of data, particularly when collected in a clinical context from an ill-defined and mobile population studied over long periods of time, are not.

These are the issues addressed in this volume. The essence of psychopharmacology is collaboration between disciplines and between workers. One collaborator must understand the details of the techniques but the other must at least understand the principles. Between them and colleagues with whom they might also be collaborating they must select from the increasing range of available techniques those that are going to eliminate their misconceptions most rapidly.

T.J. Crow

Contributors

Harry F. Baker, Chief Research Officer
David G. Cunningham Owens, Clinical Scientific Staff, and Consultant Psychiatrist, Northwick Park Hospital
Christopher D. Frith, Senior Scientific Staff
Raymond Lofthouse, Chief Technician
Frank Owen, Senior Scientific Staff
Rosalind M. Ridley, Scientific Staff, Division of Psychiatry, MRC Clinical Research Centre, Harrow, Middlesex.

Stephen J. Gamble, User Service Supervisor, Computing Services, MRC Clinical Research Centre, Harrow, Middlesex.

Alan J. Cross, Senior Scientist, ASTRA Neuroscience Research Unit, 1 Wakefield Street, London WC1.

Michael H. Joseph, Hon. Senior Lecturer in Neuroscience, MRC Scientific Staff, Departments of Psychology and Biochemistry, Institute of Psychiatry, De Crespigny Park, London SE5 8AF.

John L. Waddington, Senior Lecturer, Department of Clinical Pharmacology, Royal College of Surgeons in Ireland, St. Stephen's Green, Dublin 2.

To Anne, Sam and Polly, and to Shelagh

1 *John L. Waddington*

Psychopharmacological studies in rodents: stereotaxic intracerebral injections and behavioural assessment

1.1 Stereotaxically controlled intracerebral injections and neurotoxic lesions

There are many circumstances in which it may be advantageous to introduce very small quantities of drugs, in very small quantities of solvent,
directly into discrete areas of the central nervous system. The blood–
brain barrier and the distribution of many peripherally administered
drugs throughout virtually the whole brain are examples of some of the
factors precluding the regional localisation of any neurochemical effect
and possible resultant behavioural change(s). The development of techniques for such direct intracerebral injections has allowed much more
detailed study of the regional effects of compounds to be carried out
(Myers, 1974). However, studies utilising these procedures can be validly
interpreted only with due regard to their limitations and to the rigour of
the control procedures employed. The purpose of this section is to introduce some of these techniques and to describe some of the procedures
and problems associated with them. It is assumed that such procedures
will only be undertaken by investigators authorised and/or licensed to do
so in accordance with prevailing legislation.

Two of the most widespread uses of the intracerebral injection technique involve (a) the application of drugs into particular 'localised' cerebral
regions, with quantification of resultant neurochemical changes or behavioural response, and (b) the use of drugs that possess varieties of
neurotoxic properties allowing for the 'specific' destruction of particular
neurotransmitter systems or neuronal elements at a given site. The general aim is to introduce material directly into a circumscribed brain region
in a manner that will limit both the non-specific trauma of the procedure
and the spread of injected material away from the selected site. In the

ideal situation, use of an appropriate control will allow a valid assessment of the action of the injected material in that region.

The procedures and problems described involve stereotaxic injections directly into the anaesthetised animal. For studies in the conscious animal a guide cannula is stereotaxically implanted and attached to the animal's skull (Myers, 1971). Drug deposition is then made after recovery, via a fine injection cannula that is inserted through and directed by the guide cannula to the desired site. Most of the general principles and issues discussed in this section apply to both situations.

1.1.1 *Intracerebral injections under stereotaxic control*

1.1.1.1 *Principles and equipment.* All conventional stereotaxic frames have as their basis a carriage on the end of an arm that can be semi-micromanipulated along vernier scales in three dimensions, anterior–posterior (front to back), lateral (side to side) and dorsal–ventral (up and down) (Fig. 1.1). When combined with a restraining system to hold the anaesthetised animal's head firmly in a fixed position, via the ears (ear bars) and jaw (bite or incisor bar), the attachment of an injection unit to the carriage allows the accurate and consistent positioning of the cannula tip at designated coordinates (Fig. 1.2). Reference is usually made to a stereotaxic 'atlas' of the animal's brain which indicates the coordinates of various brain areas in a series of vertical sections through the brain serially in the anterior–posterior and lateral planes. The coordinates in such atlases are usually relative to a given reference point, sometimes the point where the tips of the ear bars (see below) meet when equally inserted along their guide channels in the absence of an animal, midpoint of the intra-aural line. Sometimes the actual reference or 'zero' point is a fixed distance from this theoretical point, to allow an even distribution of positive and negative coordinate values above and below the 'zero'. Similarly, sometimes the 'bite bar' (see below) must be set a fixed distance above or below the intra-aural line to give a particular angle of inclination of the animal's head to comply with the conventions of a given atlas. Pellegrino and Cushman (1971) have provided a detailed guide to these concepts of stereotaxis, and to the available atlases and their coordinate conventions.

The injection system itself usually involves an injection cannula fixed to the carriage on an arm of the stereotaxic frame. It should ideally be of as fine an external diameter as possible, to cause the absolute minimum of tissue damage when inserted through the brain to the desired coordinate. However, too fine a cannula will have both a greater degree of flexibility and a lack of physical resilience. With a very fine cannula (0.2 mm) great care and steadiness is required in all procedures. We have found 0.3–0.4

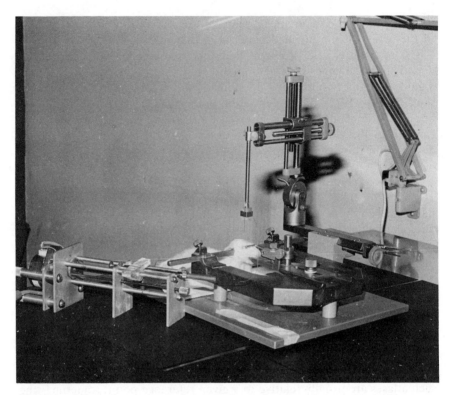

Fig. 1.1.   View of stereotaxic frame and associated equipment for intracerebral injections.

mm external diameter units to be sufficiently robust for routine work. They should be of the order of 5 cm in length and of stainless steel. The injection tip should usually be filed smooth and flat for an even outflow, though if it is desired to direct the outflow with a particular bias, e.g. diagonally, a bevelled tip can be obtained or prepared as required.

The peripheral end of the cannula unit is usually attached by a length of fine-bore flexible tubing to the delivery system. This is preferable to delivery systems with a syringe and drive attaching directly to the arm of the stereotaxic frame since the weight and dimensions of such systems create some degree of instability which can be translated into fine movements of the injection tip of the cannula. The flexible connecting tubing should be as short as possible to create the minimum of dead volume to be filled between syringe and cannula; this can be important with expensive and unstable neurotoxins, which may have to be loaded into the syringe cold from a stock solution held in an ice bucket. The tubing should, however, be of sufficient length to allow the arm of the stereotaxic frame to travel freely beyond the maximum extent likely to be required during the procedure. All joints should be carefully sealed with epoxy-resin adhesive and checked before use.

The syringe system containing the solution to be injected can be of two main types: a conventional glass-barrelled syringe with hand micrometer drive (e.g. Alga), or else a microvolume glass syringe (e.g. $1-10$ μl as required) with a slow-motion motor-driven infusor pump. Although the latter is to be preferred, the former can be rather cheaper and is in common use. Myers (1971) has reviewed several of these issues and principles.

1.1.1.2 *Setting up.* The bite bar, over which the animal's front teeth are placed, should be set at the required position, considering the conventions of the coordinate system of any stereotaxic atlas employed. The arm of the frame bearing the injection needle should be manipulated until the tip of the injection cannula is at the exact centre of the line joining the tips of the ear bars. This is most easily accomplished by bringing the ear bars together so that their points touch at the centre of the intra-aural line, and then moving each bar back (i.e. laterally) by $0.3-0.4$ mm and manipulating the needle tip into the vacated space to lie where their points previously met. This can sometimes be made easier by inserting a white card below and behind the point of intersection to improve contrast while judging the correct position. The coordinates corresponding to this position of the cannula tip can then be read from the frame and noted down. These constitute the zero reference point. It should be restated that the coordinate systems of some stereotaxic atlases may require a fixed value to be added to the coordinate in one dimension (usually the dorsal–ventral) to achieve correspondence between the cannula tip and the atlas (see above). Having obtained zero coordinates to correspond with the designated zero in the atlas, the values of the coordinates in the atlas corresponding to the desired anatomical site of the injection can then be added or subtracted (as appropriate) to those values for each dimension to derive the frame coordinate that will allow the tip to be brought ultimately to that site. The frame arm can then be moved well away from the area to allow the animal to be inserted without fear of touching the needle tip and possibly displacing it. If it is displaced during setting up or while inserting the animal, it will have to be reset.

1.1.1.3 *Anaesthesia.* It will be necessary to undertake preliminary studies to arrive at an anaesthetic paradigm that will give both sufficient depth of anaesthesia to allow the experiment to proceed humanely and a good likelihood of the animal subsequently recovering uneventfully. Use of barbiturate (e.g. sodium pentobarbitone) or volatile (e.g. halothane) anaesthetic is common. Ether can be used, but may be the method of choice only when an extremely rapid recovery is required after an intracerebral injection. It is wise not to rely on the dose or rate of delivery of anaesthetic suggested by the manufacturer's literature without preliminary study. In various strains or sizes of animal the entire spectrum of possible effects (from slight sleepyness to death) may be met at a given dose. Use of a volatile anaesthetic such as halothane may require specialised equipment for delivery, via a snout mask, and expert advice might usefully be sought. Ether may be administered initially in a jar with cotton wool attached to the top (to avoid irritating the feet) and then via a soaked and squeezed cotton wool pad placed over the snout while in the stereotaxic frame, with preliminary experiments determining the quantity and duration of its application for adequate anaesthesia. The experimenter him/herself may well be influenced by ether fumes if this open technique is employed; naturally, naked flames and hot apparatus should be removed and adequate ventilation ensured. Barbiturate anaesthesia is more straightforward but less predictable in its effect, with a low ratio between effective and lethal doses particularly in animals with respiratory tract infections. Chloral hydrate (300–400 mg/kg i.p.) may be better tolerated but may not give comparable depth of anaesthesia. In our laboratory, where respiratory tract infection appears from time to time, we have evolved the following paradigm for barbiturate anaesthesia to maximise utility and reproducibility, and to minimise carrying out surgery on animals which subsequently fail to recover. Sodium pentobarbitone (commonly used at a dose of 50–60 mg/kg) is given intraperitoneally to a group of male Sprague–Dawley rats (150–250 g) at a dose of 35–45 mg/kg. After 15–20 min, each animal is inspected for loss of righting reflex. Animals that fail to show the righting reflex are observed for rate and depth of respiration. Those breathing rapidly, in whom respiratory movements involve principally the chest and for whom a tail pinch induces a small reflex response, are selected for surgery. Where breathing is slower, deeper and perhaps irregular, involving large abdominal movements, we have found ultimate full recovery less likely. Of course, if a tail pinch produces a prominent vocal response or an attempt by the animal to right itself, anaesthesia is inadequate. In this case the animal may be used again in a few days' time; it is often possible to give a supplement of anaesthetic, but this is a risky business and no specific details can be given that will ensure a successful outcome. Immediately prior to placement in the stereotaxic frame, animals selected for surgery are given 5 mg/kg diazepam intraperitoneally. We have found that this combination of a slightly less than usual dose of barbiturate together with a benzodiazepine makes for a greater percentage of adequate anaesthesia and successful recovery when large numbers of animals are being subjected to stereotaxic surgery. *No* surgery should ever be performed under a benzodiazepine alone; the sedation and loss of righting reflex induced should not be misinterpreted as anaesthesia.

It is often the case that a pharmacological pretreatment distinct from anaesthesia is given before surgery, to influence the outcome of the intra-cerebral injection; for example, an inhibitor of noradrenaline reuptake mechanisms such as desipramine may be given to protect noradrenaline-containing neurones from the neurotoxic action of intracerebral 6-hydroxydopamine (see below). Such pretreatments may also influence anaesthesia, often increasing the effectiveness of a given anaesthetic dose and therefore increasing the likelihood of fatalities unless this is reduced. We have found a reduction of pentobarbitone dosage to 25–35 mg/kg to be required in animals pretreated with desipramine or nomifensine for the above reason (Waddington, 1980).

1.1.1.4 *The stereotaxic procedure.* Adequately anaesthetised animals must be placed accurately in the stereotaxic frame, and this is no easy business for those without experience. The principal difficulty is with the insertion of the ear bars into the auditory canal (external auditory meatus), and there is no substitute for repeated practice. We proceed as follows with a David Kopf frame. With the rat flat, back uppermost, introduce the tips of the ear bars with both hands into the auditory apertures via the ears. Manipulate and gently feel for the tips slipping into the external auditory meatus. Some idea of its position can be got by a prior visual examination of the ear. A sign of correct insertion is a characteristic 'blink' of the eyes as the ear bar tips penetrate appropriate-ly. Commercially obtained ear bars will have points shaped to limit penetration so that no permanent damage is done by this procedure. It may be tempting initially to insert the ear bars one at a time, but it will ultimately be much easier if the skill of inserting them together is ac-quired. After correct insertion, apply a gentle inward pressure and lift the animal so that the ear bars may be slotted into their guide channels in the frame. It is important that retaining-securing bolts have been previously opened to allow the bars to slip easily into these guides. When they are placed in their channels, the securing bolts must be tightened one at a time with fingers other than the forefinger and thumb usually involved in holding the ear bars. The position of the head and ear bars in the lateral plane is of no importance at this stage. When initially acquiring these techniques it may be tempting to seek the assistance of a second pair of hands. Ultimately the operator should aspire to performing the procedure unaided and only repeated practice will allow this.

. When the ear bars have been secured without the head slipping from restraint, one finger of each hand should be placed on the end of each ear bar and the bolts should then be released, with other fingers, under a slight inward pressure. Maintaining this inward pressure, the head and ear bars can be shifted from side to side in the guide channels to allow the head to be placed in a central position on the intra-aural line by reference to the scales on the ear bars and guides, and the bolts can then be resecured. It is possible to check that the ear bars are still correctly inserted by raising and lowering the animal's snout; the head should swivel smoothly about the intra-aural line only, if the bite/incisor bar is retracted sufficiently to allow free movement of the head. With the bite bar now under the snout, open the animal's mouth and place the upper incisors over it. Draw the bite bar gently back until resistance is felt and tighten the retaining screw. If the frame possesses a second bar at the head that can be lowered or screwed down on to the snout, this should be tightened only enough to grip the snout securely and hold the upper incisors in position. Should the animal vocalise or wriggle during insertion into the frame, anaesthesia is inadequate. A pad underneath the animal's body will insulate it from the cold floor of the stereotaxic frame (Fig. 1.2). A thermostatically controlled heated pad or blanket may be required in order to avoid temperature change.

1.1.1.5 *Surgical preparation.* Assuming the rat is adequately anaesthetised and correctly inserted into the frame, introduce the tip of a scalpel into the centre of the snout and draw backwards over the skull along the midline. The cut should cease at the neck, i.e. be 2.5–3 cm (1–1½ in) long. With a sharp blade the skin should separate readily to reveal the skull with a transparent, membranous covering. This periosteum should be scraped from the surface of the skull, and sufficient area exposed to allow the intracerebral injection to proceed unhindered. The skin may be held aside with retractors if necessary. The tip of the injection cannula should now be brought to just over the mid-line and the correct coordinate set in the anterior–posterior plane.

At this stage it must be decided whether the lateral coordinate should be set relative to the lateral zero of the frame or to the midline of the skull. There are advantages and disadvantages to both procedures. Use of the lateral frame zero relies on the symmetry of the skull, insertion of the ear bars to equal depths into the auditory meati and the brain lying symmetrically in the skull with its midline intersecting the centre of the intra-aural line. Reliance on the midline of the skull requires it to follow

Fig. 1.2.   Top: close-up of rat in stereotaxic frame, showing head restrained via ear bars and bite bar. The injection cannula is shown directly over the animal's head. Bottom: diagrammatic representation of the animal's head, in the same orientation as above, indicating how the injection cannula can move in three dimensions: anterior–posterior (A–P, front to back); lateral (L–L, side to side); dorsal–ventral (D–V, up and down).

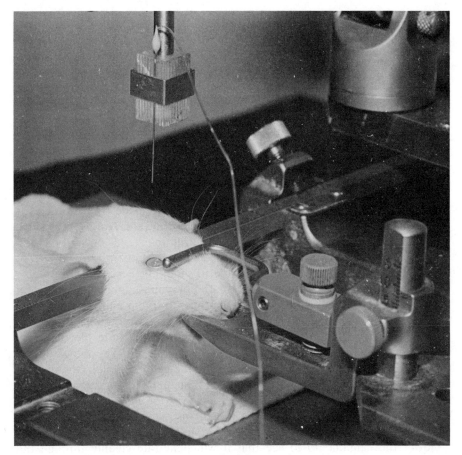

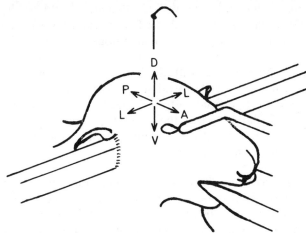

the midline of the brain, and visual observation will often show the midline of the skull to follow a meandering course. It is our practice to routinely set lateral coordinates relative to the midline of the skull. Whichever choice is made, a lateral coordinate can now be set. The cannula tip should now be above the surface of the skull and fixed in two dimensions, with only the dorsal–ventral position to be set.

The cannula tip should now be carefully lowered until it just comes in contact with the surface of the skull directly over the ultimate site of injection. If the skull has previously been wiped dry with a swab, it will now be possible to raise the cannula tip fractionally and mark with a pencil the point where its passage through the skull will be required. When so marked the injection unit can be raised safely away again. A hole of approximately 1 mm diameter should be made by hand. This is best accomplished by placing an appropriate drill (e.g. No. 57) in a small hand chuck so that only 1–1.5 mm of the drill tip extends beyond the grip of the chuck; this will prevent the drill tip penetrating into the cortex (or deeper!) when the hole has been made. It should be necessary to use only a gentle pressure on the marked spot. For young animals, say rats of 150–200 g, the skull wil be thin and fibrous; for older animals it will be a little thicker and tougher. Fluid or blood may seep from the hole unless it is within approximately 1 mm of the midline when copious bleeding may be seen from the moment the drill penetrates the skull. This indicates that the sagittal sinus, a blood vessel following the general path of the midline and lying just below the skull, has been punctured. If ruptured, bleeding will be difficult to control. Firm pressure over the hole with a swab may stem external but not internal bleeding. This problem should be avoided if at all possible. Having prepared a hole through the skull, carefully lower the cannula tip to see that it will penetrate cleanly through the hole, and that it has not been drilled off-centre; if this is the case, the injection unit is raised again and the hole is carefully widened with the drill to ensure clean passage. The membranous lining of the brain (dura) must now be pierced to allow subsequent penetration into the brain. A fine needle (25 or 26 gauge) with the lower 1–2 mm bent at right angles will be useful for this, as the bend stops over-zealous movements from causing more than superficial cortical damage by again limiting the depth of penetration. Failure to pierce the dura adequately will mean the needle tip will catch on it, with possible deformation of the brain surface by compression and of the cannula itself.

1.1.1.6 *The intracerebral injection.* Assuming appropriate surgical preparation to allow clean passage of the cannula into the brain, the injection system must now be filled. With a large syringe barrel, this can be done conventionally taking extra special care to ensure that the system is free from air bubbles and that material is ejected smoothly from the cannula tip *before* intracerebral insertion. With microsyringe barrels, say 1–10 μl in a microinfusor pump unit, it is more difficult, and is most easily done by fitting a 1 ml conventional syringe with a very fine (26 gauge) needle that can be inserted into the plunger end of the microsyringe. The system can be filled in this way and the plunger replaced. Again, the system should be checked for smooth ejection of material from the cannula tip before introduction into the brain.

With the cannula tip wiped free of any external fluid from setting up and filling, the injection unit can now be slowly lowered into the brain until the desired coordinate is reached. There are no empirical data on the effects of rate of passage through the brain in producing non-specific tissue damage. However, it seems reasonable to make this as slow and steady as is convenient. The scale indicating the vertical coordinate should be observed carefully in order not to overrun the desired site, as drawing back will vacate a space into which injected material can flow away from the desired location. With the cannula tip in the desired location, the delivery can now be made. When the delivery has been finished, the cannula must be maintained in position for a while to allow diffusion of injected material into tissue. The volume and rate of delivery and needle retention are important factors which will be covered in detail below. Thereafter the injection unit can be slowly raised out of the brain. Immediately the cannula tip becomes free, some injection fluid should be ejected out on to a swab placed on the head. This is to get rid of any blood or biological fluids which may have diffused or been taken up into the cannula tip. If they are allowed to remain, they may congeal or dry and thus block the delivery system. Fluid seeping from the hole in the skull will not necessarily be injected material.

1.1.1.7 *Surgical completion.* The arm of the stereotaxic frame bearing the injection unit can now be moved away from the skull and the animal freed by releasing first the bite bar and snout restraint and then the ear bars. The wound may be closed by suture or with autoclips. Adequate suturing will require considerable practice, preferably under guidance from someone with experience in either the animal or clinical operating theatre. We routinely close a 2.5–3 cm wound with four autoclips (small, 9 mm) inserted with an automatically reloading applicator. The edges of the wound should be brought closely together and the applicator brought vertically down so that the join lies between the teeth of the clip. The first clip is applied at the anterior extent of the wound and three further clips are distributed over its remaining length, with the final clip closing the posterior extent. Inspectors of the government agency controlling animal experiments in the United Kingdom (the Home Office) take the informal view that not more than four autoclips should be applied to close wounds of this length, and that they should not be kept in position for longer than 3 weeks. If survival to or beyond this time is contemplated, autoclips can be removed with the complementary extracting tool or a combination of wire cutters and forceps; light ether anaesthesia or sedation with a benzodiazepine will facilitate autoclip removal if these treatments are thought not to prejudice experiments in hand.

While recovering from anaesthesia after wound closure and removal from the frame, the animal should be kept warm. This is more important if barbiturate anaesthesia has been used. Placing the animal in a cage on bedding such as clean, dry sawdust or fine shavings, with a lamp containing a low-wattage bulb held 30–45 cm over the cage, will usually suffice.

In some institutes it is routine to give prophylactic antibiotics to maximise the likelihood of safe outcome from surgery. Other institutes may forbid this routinely for fear of ultimately generating resistant organisms with serious attendant problems. It is our practice not to give antibiotics routinely after surgery. Antibiotics should be used only when veterinary officers may consider it required for humanitarian reasons on a strictly individual basis. In such circumstances they are more likely to require the animal to be sacrificed. It is a wise goal in the long run to do everything possible to help keep infective organisms, especially resistant strains, out of the animal house, even if this means the loss or sacrifice of a few (or several) animals.

1.1.2 *Problems and technical considerations*

Some minor problems and complications that may be encountered have been referred to previously. Considered here are problems that appear to be more fundamental to the overall procedure and its use in obtaining valid results.

1.1.2.1 *Relationship of the stereotaxic atlas to the anatomy of the animal.*

Stereotaxic atlases are usually derived from a fixed number of animals of a particular sex and size, taken from a particular strain. It should cause no surprise that what is true about the anatomy of a 150 g female Wistar rat may not be true of a 200 g male Sprague–Dawley counterpart (Pellegrino and Cushman, 1971). Although the general anatomical relationships will of course hold for almost all rodent subjects, the same cannot be said for the precise quantitative details of the relative locations of specific, discrete brain areas. A knowledge of these quantitative details is vital for stereotaxic work, but they may differ even between subjects drawn from the same strain and of the same size and sex. These differences may arise because of general biological variability in cerebral anatomy or because of variability in auditory canal or jaw formation controlling the position of fixation in the stereotaxic frame.

Some general idea of the relationship between coordinate anatomy in the stereotaxic atlas and cerebral anatomy in animals of the species, sex and size to hand may be obtained from obligatory preliminary experiments. In these, the injection unit is lowered to the coordinates selected direct from the atlas, in several animals. The animals may be quickly killed, perhaps by giving an overdose of anaesthetic prior to surgery, and immediately processed for histological verification of the location of the tip of the cannula. No specific detailed histological procedures are given, as they are beyond the scope of this text. An introductory guide (e.g. Wolf, 1971) or, better still, an expert histopathologist should be consulted for advice. If such histological studies are carried out immediately after surgery, the needle tract will be found to be filled with blood, making it easier to follow and locate the ultimate site of the tip. This 'marker' will be degraded and disappear with time after death, making the location of cannula tracts less easy. In a group of several animals it may be found that the sites of cannula tips approximate closely to that desired on the basis of the coordinates chosen. If so, the study proper may begin. It may, however, be that the location of the cannula tips may be consistently some distance away from that desired. If this is the case, a compensating factor must be applied to the atlas coordinate to give better correspondence with the cerebral anatomy of the subjects used.

1.1.2.2 *Volume and rate of intracerebral infusion.* The delivery of a large volume of injected material directly into brain tissue is clearly a non-physiological event. Two problems associated with the procedure are therefore tissue damage, by way of mechanical displacement via the cannula or the bulk of injection, and spread of injected material away from the desired site by diffusion through tissue, thus confounding relationships between site of injection and site of action. Cannula damage can be minimised by the use of the finest cannula appropriate, as considered earlier. The other artefacts can be minimised, but not eliminated, by using the smallest possible volume infused at the slowest possible rate. We are dealing here with volumes in the microlitre or fractional microlitre range, infused over a period of at least 1 min.

The choice of absolute volume and rate of delivery are governed to some extent by the area of the anatomical region into which that delivery is to be made. Larger volumes, say $1-4$ μl, can be delivered into a relatively large structure such as the striatum, where they may have the paradoxical advantage of diffusing away from the injection site and thus enabling some, but not all, materials to reach striatal areas distant from the point of delivery. Larger volumes also allow lower concentrations of injected material to be maintained; this can be an advantage where non-specific cytotoxic actions of drugs are concentration related. However, for accurate placement and confinement of injected material, smaller volumes must be preferred. For injections into structures of reduced dimensions, such as the nucleus accumbens, a volume of 1 μl must be considered maximal. Even this volume is felt by some workers to be so large as to preclude valid studies. Where one is trying to dissociate effects obtained from closely related sites, such as individual hypothalamic areas, things become even more problematical. We have found it possible to dissociate drug effects in structures separated by as little as 0.5 mm, using an injection volume of 1 μl into the zona reticulata and zona compacta of the rat substantia nigra (Waddington and Longden, 1977; Waddington, 1978). However, such anatomical dissociation may well have been more marked had smaller volumes been used. Myers (1971) and James and Starr (1978) have carefully studied the differential effects of varying injection volumes infused into such closely related sites. A volume of 0.2–0.5 μl might be considered an acceptable compromise, with 0.1–0.2 μl being difficult to eject from a conventional cannula without recourse to ultra-fine stainless-steel tubing or glass capillaries. For routine work we regularly use a volume of 0.5–1.0 μl for drug injections into discrete brain structures, and 1–4 μl for injections of neurotoxins to induce 'localised' lesions.

The rate of delivery is influenced by the apparatus used for that delivery. Slow-motion microinfusion is to be preferred, but only a hand micrometer-driven syringe may be available. In the latter case it is quite a common practice to deliver a 1 μl volume as slowly as possible over a period of the order of 5 s, and allow the injection cannula to remain in position for a further 55 s to enable the material to diffuse into the surrounding tissue. If a large volume is required, this process can be repeated in 1 μl steps until the desired total volume is delivered. However, continuous infusion by a motor-driven, slow-motion micro-delivery system is to be preferred. Here a microsyringe (1–10 μl) is placed in an apparatus which automatically drives the plunger down the syringe barrel at a very slow but constant rate, expelling material extremely gradually into tissue surrounding the cannula tip. There are few quantitative studies in this area, but it seems reasonable to assume that the slower the rate of infusion, the less marked the resultant tissue damage might be. Infusion rates of 1 μl per 10–15 min or longer have been used, but in particular cases they may be inappropriate for routine work. We regularly use an infusion rate of 1 μl/min via a slow-motion pump.

When the intracerebral injection has been completed, the cannula should be retained in position for an additional period to allow complete diffusion of material. This is to reduce its retrograde flow along the needle tract when it is withdrawn, thus eliminating loss of material from the desired site and widespread dispersion over the brain. Ideally this period should also be as long as is practicable, and periods of up to

10 min have been used. For no empirically determined reason we have regularly used a 1 min retention period and have found this appropriate for routine work. Periods of less than 1 min should not be considered.

1.1.2.3 *Injection vehicle.* It is important to emphasise that the effects of an intracerebral injection of a drug may not be equated with an action of that drug *unless* comparisons are made with a control group receiving identical injection only of the fluid in which that drug was dissolved. Physiological saline, distilled water or phosphate-buffered saline have all been used for water-soluble substances, and a variety of acids or organic solvents for insoluble material. Acidic or organic solvents/solutions can have marked effects in their own right without requiring the addition of any drug substance and their use should be avoided if possible. Attempts to neutralise acidic solutions to physiological pH are not always successful and may result in the dissolved substance coming out of solution as a precipitate. Sometimes it may be possible to obtain a water-soluble derivative of the required drug or a water-soluble member of the same pharmacological class. We were once interested in injecting benzodiazepines intracerebrally; diazepam could be dissolved only in an acidic solution and gave a marked pharmacological effect that was exactly reproduced by identical injections of the acid vehicle alone! Benzodiazepine effects were, however, obtained by turning to the water-soluble agents chlordiazepoxide HCl and flurazepam HCl. We routinely use 0.9% physiological saline as our injection vehicle, adding other ingredients according to characteristics of the particular drug.

Much use has been made of intracerebral injections of the monoamine neurotoxins 6-hydroxydopamine (6-OHDA) and 5,6- and 5,7-dihydroxytryptamine (5,6- and 5,7-DHT). These hydroxylated analogues of monoamine neurotransmitters are widely used to induce 'selective' chemical lesions of catecholamine-or indoleamine-containing neurones respectively, by their intracerebral application on to the relevant cell bodies, axons or terminals (Baumgarten *et al.*, 1977; Breese and Cooper, 1977). They are rapidly oxidised at neutral pH and require addition of an antioxidant to the injection vehicle. We have routinely used ascorbic acid for this purpose, at concentrations of 1 mg/ml for 6-OHDA and 0.2 mg/ml for 5,6- and 5,7-DHT. On the basis of studies referred to later, we feel the concentration for 6-OHDA could be reduced to at least that used for the dihydroxytryptamines. Such solutions should be protected from light and held on ice until required for syringe filling. We routinely do this for all materials we inject intracerebrally. Even though more than a single injection can often be made from our filled microsyringe, we also empty our syringe after each animal and refill freshly for the next, to obviate any possible degradation of the material. The most widely used concentrations for the neurotoxins are 2–4 $\mu g/\mu l$ in a total volume of 2–4 μl for 6-OHDA and 1–2 $\mu g/\mu l$ in the same volume for 5,6- and 5,7-DHT. We have used 8 $\mu g/4$ μl for 6-OHDA and 5 $\mu g/4$ μl for the dihydroxytryptamines routinely (Waddington and Crow, 1979a). Mention has been made of the use of pretreatments with drugs to influence or enhance the 'specificity' of action of monoamine neurotoxins, and further details can be found elsewhere (Baumgarten *et al.*, 1977; Breese and Cooper, 1977; Waddington, 1980). The ability of such pretreatments to potentiate depth of anaesthesia with barbiturates, as described earlier, should not be forgotten.

In addition to the desired pharmacological properties of the vehicle solution, it can disrupt tissue function in its own right. Both Wolfarth *et al.* (1977) and ourselves (Waddington and Crow, 1979b) have found intracerebral injections of saline containing ascorbic acid (and to a lesser extent saline alone) to induce both behavioural and neurochemical changes. In other instances we have found reproducible behavioural responses to intracerebral saline (Waddington, 1978). Such results have at least two major implications. First, results with drugs delivered in such vehicles can only be validly interpreted when compared with those of a full vehicle control injection; it is not sufficient, as is sometimes done, to lower the needle to the designated site but not include actual injection of vehicle. Secondly, vehicle-injected animals cannot be considered 'normal' controls unless shown in the test situation (neurochemical or behavioural, or both) to be indistinguishable from ordinary intact rats not subjected to any surgical procedure.

1.1.2.4 *Unblocking the injection cannula.* During the course of a single or several intracerebral injections the cannula may become blocked. Congealed biological fluids are a common cause, and steps to minimise the likelihood of this occurring have been discussed earlier. Small pieces of biological material or environmental contaminants are also capable of blocking a fine cannula. One advantage of emptying our microsyringe after each animal has been injected is that any blockages become readily apparent. If ejection of material is not checked for each animal when several animals are injected from the same syringe after filling, then a blockage may become apparent only because of a surprising lack of effect of the procedure; the material may, in fact, have exited through leaking joints or via the syringe plunger under increased internal pressure. If the syringe cannot be unblocked by attempting to force a full syringe of physiological saline through the system under moderate hand pressure, a length of very fine wire, e.g. fuse wire, can be poked into the cannula tip. This may dislodge blocking material and allow it to be ejected under pressure. This method will be less appropriate if the blockage is distal to the cannula, e.g. within the microsyringe outflow. In such a case it is often possible to remove the syringe plunger, fill a separate 1 ml syringe with saline and attach to it a wide-bore needle. If this can be slipped over the cannula tip, saline can be forced in reverse through the microsyringe plunger channel. We have found two procedures to give some protection against blockages. Expelling some injection material immediately after raising the cannula from the brain, ejecting substances incorporated into the cannula tip that may congeal, has been noted above. Furthermore, scrupulous cleanliness should be observed when the microsyringe plunger is withdrawn for filling (e.g. it should not be placed on a possibly contaminated bench, and the needle used for refilling the syringe should be wiped clean before each use).

1.1.2.5 *Histological and neurochemical verification of injection.* For reasons noted earlier it cannot be assumed that injections delivered under particular stereotaxic coordinates will arrive in the animal at the anatomical site corresponding to these coordinates in the atlas. The location of intracerebral injections must be verified in some way before results can be validly interpreted. Such verification can be histological, neurochemical or both.

Histological verification seeks to confirm anatomically that the tip of the injection cannula did indeed terminate at the desired location for each animal. Results from incorrectly injected animals must be discarded. In one instance we found intracerebral injections to be consistently misplaced because a stereotaxic coordinate had been set 1 mm in error; the lack of effect at this site was subsequently used as an unplanned-for anatomical control group. During routine work where many uniform animals are being subjected to identical surgery, some workers verify their injections by sampling. One of every six, say, may be taken for histology to ensure that nothing has gone amiss. As noted previously, no specific detailed histological procedures are given here. Someone with considerable practical experience should be consulted, not because the techniques are intrinsically difficult, but rather because they are most easily acquired by expert demonstration rather than by anecdotal instruction or from a manual that may assume too much prior knowledge. Such histological examination will additionally reveal not only the position of the cannula tip but also the extent of any tissue damage or pathology in the area surrounding the tip that may have been induced by the physical bulk of the material injected. This is a useful form of validation in instances where the material injected is neurotoxic and is associated with a characteristic profile of pathological changes. An example would be the excitatory amino acid analogue, kainic acid (KA), which has been proposed to 'selectively' induce degeneration of neuronal cell bodies near to the cannula tip, while sparing nerve axons and terminals in that area (McGeer *et al.*, 1978). For this compound, validation is not simply a matter of confirming the site of injection but of confirming the nature and regional specificity of the localised pathological changes induced. Confirmation of typical patterns of cell loss (McGeer *et al.*, 1978) and their confinement to the desired area can be obtained using straightforward techniques of histological examination.

An alternative, or sometimes complementary, technique is neurochemical validation. Here, characteristic neurochemical changes after intracerebral injection of a particular substance might be sought, for example loss of striatal dopamine content after application of 6-OHDA on to cell bodies, axons or terminals of the nigrostriatal dopaminergic pathway. Using this technique, specificity of action can also be assessed, for example by assaying the content of striatal 5-hydroxytryptamine after 6-OHDA lesions of DA axons (see Table 1.1). In doing this we have noted small but significant reductions in striatal 5-HT content after 6-OHDA (Waddington and Crow, 1979b). It is important to consider here the whole issue of the specificity of action of such monoamine neurotoxins, as a wide-ranging debate since their introduction has failed to produce a consensus opinion on this (Breese and Cooper, 1977; Waddington and Crow, 1979a,b). They remain in widespread use and if these limitations are realised they remain tools of remarkable utility. The same strategy can be used with KA. Rather than confirming the localisation of its neurotoxic action by histopathological examination, characteristic neurochemical changes resultant from pathological changes can be studied. For example, following intrastriatal KA the loss of striatal perikarya is reflected in reduced activities of several marker enzymes such as glutamic acid decarboxylase and cholineacetyltransferase in that area (McGeer *et al.*, 1978). This can provide a useful validation of a successful lesion. We have been able to dissociate the action of KA in the striatum from that in the closely related nucleus accumbens using this procedure (Waddington and Cross, 1978). However, as more detailed examinations of the pathological and neurochemical sequelae of intracerebral KA have proceeded, so more doubts are raised about its absolute specificity of action for neuronal cell bodies in a given area (McGeer *et al.*, 1978; Wuerthele *et al.*, 1978). Also, its intracerebral application has been associated with distant neuronal damage, not only by diffusion but also by propagation of convulsive neuronal activity; this can be limited by a pretreatment with diazepam (Ben-Ari *et al.*, 1979; Cross and Waddington, 1981). Both of these issues should be born in mind when interpreting results obtained using intracerebral KA. The use of a further excitatory amino acid analogue, ibotenic acid, has been proposed as a similar but superior lesioning tool (Schwarcz *et al.*, 1979).

It is sometimes tempting to resort to behavioural or functional validation of the site of action of intracerebrally administered drugs. Here the experimenter assumes that because a characteristic behavioural response to an intracerebral injection is reliably observed, similar to that described in previous histologically validated studies, the injection site must be correct. This may or may not follow. The injection may not be exactly in the required location but material may be diffusing to the ultimately desired site to induce that effect. In these circumstances, a changed time course or intensity of effect will induce unnecessary biological variability into overall responses. They may be modulated by such actions in closely related regions with similar results. Such circumstances call for serial sampling for histological verification as a minimum precaution. Despite this, certain behavioural responses have been noted to predict empirically at least the general accuracy of an intracerebral injection, and this is especially true for neurotoxins. For example, in the very earliest stages of recovery from anaesthesia, two of the most widely used neurotoxins produce characteristic behavioural patterns when injected unilaterally into the nigrostriatal system. Such injections are often made in connection with the so-called rotating circling or turning rat model that is widely used for the assessment of drug action on this system (Pycock, 1980). 6-OHDA is associated with postural asymmetry characterised by stumbling forwards with the body curved towards the side receiving the intra-

Table 1.1. Neurochemical sequelae of control procedures and 6-OHDA. (From Waddington and Crow, 1979b.)

Procedure	*DA striatum*	*5-HT striatum*	*NA cortex*	*5-HT cortex*
None	+17.9	+6.4	—	—
Needle only	−10.7	−2.8	—	—
Saline	−18.5	−6.9	−4.9	+7.9
Saline + 0.2 mg/ml ascorbate	+22.1*	−13.8	−5.1	+0.6
Saline + 1.0 mg/ml ascorbate	−21.4**	−11.7	−10.0	+1.1
6-OHDA 8 μg + 1.0 mg/ml ascorbate	−83.7***	−23.7**	−92.3***	−8.7

Regional concentrations of dopamine (DA), noradrenaline (NA) and 5-hydroxytryptamine (5-HT), following various control procedures and 6-OHDA. Results are expressed as percentage change in injected compared with non-injected hemisphere, using a site in the medial forebrain bundle and an injection volume of 4 μl. Values are means of 3–9 samples. Significant differences between injected and non-injected hemispheres: *, $p < 0.05$; **, $p < 0.01$; ***, $p < 0.001$ (*t*-test).

cerebral injection during recovery. Intrastriatal KA is associated with marked rotation about the long axis of the body (barrel rotation) and directed away from the side receiving the injection, under similar conditions. Although such behavioural signs can usefully predict which animals have been successfully lesioned and can be used for further work, those proceeded with must be ultimately subjected to neurochemical or histological validation. Also, in some circumstances failure to show a supposed characteristic sign may result in the unwitting rejection of important data, perhaps from an animal showing no effect because of an interesting interaction with two closely related but opposing processes.

1.1.2.6 *Clarification of some further artefacts.* It may sometimes be observed that, when a substance is injected intracerebrally, effects are noted only at extremely high concentrations. This may reflect the intrinsically low potency of the drug or its rapid metabolism at and diffusion away from the injection site. If the material is being enzymatically degraded, a pretreatment with an inhibitor of that enzyme may be useful if available, e.g. a monoamine oxidase inhibitor prior to intracerebral injections of monoamine neurotransmitters. However, the effects of such pretreatments themselves must be considered. In some cases, the effectiveness of a drug only at higher concentrations may be indicative of a non-specific process such as membrane stabilising or local anaesthetic action. The possibility of such an effect should not be overlooked, and comparisons with similar injections of a known local anaesthetic may be useful in some cases. However, inhibition of cellular activity may be mediated by a genuine pharmacological action, e.g. activation of physiological inhibitory processes. Therefore, reproduction of an effect by a local anaesthetic need not necessarily indicate such an action for the drug under investigation.

When a drug produces a particular effect on intracerebral injection into a given site, this action may be mediated by diffusion to an anatomically related area. Speed of onset of acute effects may be an occasional indicator, but it should not be relied upon and is not appropriate for agents acting more progressively, e.g. monoamine neurotoxins. Making similar injections into surrounding tissue areas will enable the most sensitive site to be detected and isolated. Where necessary, the extent of diffusion of radiolabelled drug or analogue may be estimated by autoradiography. ^{14}C-Neurotransmitters have been used to estimate the spread of intracerebrally injected compounds and analogues under particular injection parameters (Myers and Hoch, 1978). Similar injections of dyes have been made, but it is not possible to equate the spread of dyestuffs reliably with the extent of tissue diffusion of drugs themselves (Myers, 1971).

It should not be overlooked that many other factors, unconnected with the nature of the actual procedures employed, can influence the sequelae of intracerebral injections of drugs. For example, the age of animal used can influence the extent of neurotoxicity seen following intracerebral KA (Gaddy *et al.*, 1979). There may also be strain differences in responsivity to stereotaxically injected neurotoxins (Sanberg *et al.*, 1979). Such effects may confound comparisons between studies just as much as any differences in the injection parameters utilised.

1.2 Assessment of rodent behaviour in relation to dopaminergic processes

Inspection of any introductory text on behavioural pharmacology (e.g. Iversen and Iversen, 1981) will indicate the wide and still growing scope of the topic. Some of the many areas in which the behavioural effects of drugs have been particularly studied include conditioned behaviour, group or social behaviour, and the motor behaviour of single animals. It is with this last area that this section will principally concern itself. Although many classes of drugs acting on the CNS are widely known to induce characteristic changes in rodent motor behaviour, the way in which such effects are assessed and quantified has received far less systematic investigation. Studies from several laboratories purporting to examine the same behavioural phenomena will often be found to utilise differing techniques, procedures and criteria of effects, thus confounding their comparison and interpretation. Thus, tissue concentrations of a neurotransmitter such as dopamine may be assayed by several different techniques (e.g. radioenzymatic, HPLC, GC–MS; see Chapter 4) with the reasonable expectation that comparable results will usually be found. However, when considering the assessment of the behavioural effects of a drug which directly (e.g. apomorphine) or indirectly (e.g. amphetamine) activates dopaminergic systems in the brain, we are dealing with variables that lend themselves less readily to such 'objective' quantification. To illustrate these general problems, we will take as an example the phenomenon of stereotyped behaviour (or stereotypy) induced by dopaminergic drugs, one of the most widely studied syndromes in psychopharmacology.

1.2.1 *Assessment of stereotyped behaviour*
1.2.1.1 *The concept of stereotypy.* If we place a rat singly in an observation cage and simply look at its behaviour for a short while, then several behaviours will be commonly noted. Such animals will usually exhibit appreciable amounts of sniffing, and may locomote about the apparatus and rear up, usually at the walls and corners, to direct sniffing over wide areas of the cage. These behaviours commonly appear in bursts that are punctuated by interpolated periods of stillness, defecation and poss-

ibly grooming. Such a profile of behaviours could be interpreted as 'exploratory' or 'investigatory' behaviour in a novel environment. After being in such a cage for some while, these bursts of 'exploratory/ investigatory' behaviour commonly become less frequent and will, over a period of 15–30 min, eventually decline. After rather longer periods, of 1 h or more, even bursts of sniffing from a stationary position may cease and the animal becomes still and quiescent. This is commonly referred to as a process of habituation to the novel environment. Note that unless consumatory behaviour is the specific subject of study, access to food and water is usually denied during such observation periods.

If a dopaminergic drug such as apomorphine is now given to such quiescent animals, in comparison with parallel animals given vehicle alone a characteristic 'activation' of behaviour is usually seen. A certain element of behaviour, or specific combinations or sequences of behaviour, come to be performed in a repetitive and seemingly inappropriate and purposeless manner, i.e. stereotyped behaviour/stereotypy. In the rat such elements include sniffing, locomotion, rearing, biting, licking and gnawing. It is important to note that the behaviours manifested in this way include some that can readily be seen spontaneously and episodically in normal, undrugged animals in situations such as the 'exploratory/ investigatory' sequence described above. However, it is the continuous performance of such behaviour(s) in so repetitive, invariant and seemingly purposeless manner, to the exclusion of other 'normal' elements of behaviour, that is the hallmark of stereotypy. The topic has been the subject of a recent comprehensive review (Robbins and Sahakian, 1981).

1.2.1.2 *Early stereotypy rating scales.* It was originally thought that the manifestation of these behaviours reflected a dose-dependent effect of such drugs on a unitary system of the brain; the stereotypies of sniffing, locomotion and rearing thought to be preferentially induced by lower doses were referred to as low-intensity features of stereotypy, and biting, licking and gnawing, commonly seen with higher doses, were referred to as high-intensity features. On this basis, simple rating scales have been, and still are, extensively used to quantify visually observed behaviour after drug challenge; the ratings represent a series of mutually exclusive categories of behaviour that were considered to reflect the increasing intensity of stereotypy (Table 1.2).

Such rating scales rely on the subjective judgement of an observer, and it is mandatory that he/she is 'blind' to (i.e. unaware of) the differing drug treatments/histories of each animal. A major problem here is that different observers may make differing subjective judgements of what constitutes a brief episode of sniffing as opposed to no stereotypy (i.e. transition between scores 0 and 1), bearing in mind that some normal

Table 1.2. Stereotypy rating scale. (From Costall *et al.* (1972).)

Score	Definition
0	The appearance of animals is the same as saline-treated rats
1	Discontinuous sniffing, constant exploratory activity
2	Continuous sniffing, periodic exploratory activity
3	Continuous sniffing, discontinuous biting, gnawing or licking. Very brief periods of locomotor activity
4	Continuous biting or licking; no exploratory activity

Note: In common use, some of the qualifying descriptions in this scale are ignored, i.e. 0 = normal; 1 = continuous locomotor activity, discontinuous sniffing; 2 = discontinuous locomotor activity, continuous sniffing; 3 = discontinuous biting, licking and gnawing; 4 = continuous biting, licking or gnawing.

animals readily sniff spontaneously even when habituated to the test apparatus for some while. Similar problems arise over defining boundaries between very frequent episodes of behaviours, sniffing or biting, and their continuous performance. A second difficulty is that such a scale is relatively insensitive to specific behaviours such as locomotion and rearing. Their omission from such scales in common use (see footnote to Table 1.2) seems to stem from the belief that sniffing and biting are the principal indicators of dose-dependent 'activation' of unitary forebrain dopamine systems. It may be that certain neurochemical processes distinguish an animal that is sniffing while stationary from one that is sniffing while locomoting and from another contemporaneously rearing. Such qualitative differences may be important behavioural indicators of specific drug effects that are overlooked using such scales.

1.2.1.3 *More recent stereotypy rating scales.* Some of these problems have been addressed by devising scales that cover a greater range of behaviours and with more explicit descriptions of the criteria for each category (Table 1.3).

Such expanded scales have certain advantages. They address the issue of distinguishing between the simple occurrence of a behaviour (i.e. scores 0 vs. 1) and whether that behaviour is being manifested in a stereotyped manner, e.g. transitions between scores of 1, 2 and 3. A second issue addressed by such a revised scale is that of the circumstances in which a stereotyped behaviour is being emitted, e.g. is stereotyped sniffing manifested during locomotion or rearing, or in a stationary, fixated position? The criteria for a score of 3 on the above scale implicitly requires the presence of locomotion and/or rearing, at least to some degree, to direct designated activities such as sniffing over different areas

Table 1.3.   Stereotypy Rating Scale. (From Creese and Iversen (1973).)

Score	Definition
0	Asleep or stationary
1	Active
2	Predominantly active but with bursts of stereotyped sniffing or rearing
3	Stereotyped activity such as sniffing along a fixed path in the cage
4	Stereotyped sniffing or rearing maintained in one location
5	Stereotyped behaviour in one location with bursts of gnawing or licking
6	Continuous gnawing or licking of cage bars

of the cage. Conversely, a score of 4 implicitly requires locomotion to be absent, such that stereotypy is maintained in one fixed position. Such criteria imply that fixation of stereotypy to one position reflects a higher intensity of response and, conversely, that the presence of locomotion and rearing reflect a lower intensity. A corollary of the above is that features such as locomotion and gnawing/licking are assumed to be unlikely to occur contemporaneously.

Unfortunately, recent studies have indicated certain circumstances in which these assumptions appear to be invalid. Thus Fray *et al.* (1980), making detailed repeated observations and using a wide range of apomorphine doses, have noted concurrent locomotion and gnawing. We have seen this composite occasionally, and have reported that such 'paradoxical' combinations of behaviours may be even more likely to occur when dopaminergic systems have been influenced by long-term phenothiazine neuroleptic treatment (Gamble and Waddington, 1981). We have also noted that during certain long-term phenothiazine treatments normal locomotor responses to apomorphine can be markedly and selectively potentiated (Waddington *et al.*, 1982). As a score of 3 would be appropriate for both circumstances (i.e. stereotyped sniffing either with a 'normal' degree of locomotion or with profoundly heightened locomotion obvious to the eye), criteria for this score are insensitive to such phenomena. Thus simple reliance on such scales, especially by an inexperienced observer, may fail to quantify these distinctions. A related problem can occur if a particular pharmacological pretreatment causes apomorphine to selectively induce profound stereotyped hyperlocomotion and sniffing, while in corresponding non-pretreated animals the response to the same apomorphine dose fulfils criteria for a score of 4. Here, marked potentiation of locomotion causes sniffing to be distributed away from any fixed location, i.e. score 3. Thus, for similar levels of sniffing, a *heightened* level of locomotion would be quantified as a *reduced* stereotypy score using the scale alone. Such behaviours are better recorded as individual categories, as described later.

It is therefore clear that, by relying on stereotypy rating scales alone, useful information may be lost or misquantified, and incorrect assumptions may be made concerning the drug effects and cerebral processes investigated. The two principal alternatives investigated over the past few years involve (a) automated assessment, and (b) improved visual observation techniques unrelated to rating scales.

1.2.2 *Automated assessment of behaviour*

1.2.2.1 *General issues.* It is not the purpose of this section to review the various running wheels, jiggle cages, photocell cages and capacitive-inductive apparatuses previously advocated for 'objective' measurement of gross, undifferentiated 'activities'. Robbins (1977) has critically analysed several modes of assessment, and Ljungberg (1978) has reported systematic, comparative studies of the effects of apomorphine using two such automatic registration devices (photocell vs. capacitative–inductive) with contemporaneous stereotypy ratings by scale. The conclusion of this latter author bears repeating:

> The results show that motor activity cannot be regarded as a simple or homogeneous behaviour that is reliably measured in conventional activity boxes. It is an undescriptive measure consisting of an artificial summation of those components of behaviour that affect the movement-detecting device in the particular box which is used. (Ljungberg, 1978, p. 191)

More sophisticated monitoring devices have been developed which allow the experimenter to set varying levels and/or modes of detection that are claimed to 'select' certain elements of behaviour for quantification. When compared with direct visual observation by rating scale in animals given dopaminergic drugs, they appear to represent some advance over their earlier, less sophisticated counterparts. However, their limited additional resolving power does not really extend to the multiple components of stereotyped behaviour (Ljungberg, 1978; Tyler and Tessel, 1979).

1.2.2.2 *Improved techniques.* Faced with such problems there are two ways of pursuing further the goal of automated assessment. The first is to design an apparatus that will both effectively limit the range of behaviours emitted and allow detection only of the desired response. Thus Olpe (1978) has described a system for the automated quantification of apomorphine-induced gnawing. This entails physical restraint of the animal to limit competing behaviours; the only other behaviours noted, but not detected by the apparatus, being sniffing and licking. Such a device artificially constrains the animal and the results so obtained in relation to gnawing cannot be generalised to the unrestrained animal in a visual observation cage. The apparatus was specifically designed to favour manifestation of gnawing to apomorphine, and it will be necessary to note below that physical features of cages and apparatus can be important determinants of the qualitative nature of the response(s) observed (response topography). Redgrave *et al.* (1982) have briefly reviewed this topic and have described a more refined apparatus which does not entail physical restraint. However, it was specifically designed to facilitate the expression and detection of gnawing rather than other forms of stereotypy. The small cage area chosen would restrict (but not eliminate) locomotion and rearing; licking was observed occasionally and no mention is made of other forms of stereotyped behaviour. Again, it may not be possible to generalise the results so obtained to an animal in a less constrained situation where other behaviours can be manifested.

An alternative approach to the automated assessment of behaviour has been studied by Ljungberg and Ungerstedt (1978a). Rather than develop an apparatus to selectively facilitate the expression and detection of one form of stereotyped behaviour, they have sought to develop an open-field device capable of detecting and quantifying each of eight classes of behaviour with the minimum of constraints on the animal. In a complex apparatus, various modes of detection were used over areas of the open field and the resultant signals were processed by microcomputer to derive the following parameters: undifferentiated activity; total locomotion; forward locomotion; hole count and hole time (relating to the number and duration of insertions of the animal's head into a series of 2.5 cm diameter holes distributed over the floor of the cage); corner count and corner time (relating to the number and duration of episodes of behaviour directed into cage corners, as opposed to elsewhere); gnawing (almost always performed on the edge of the holes, in the absence of any other appropriate feature of the apparatus). This sophisticated (and expensive) apparatus has been used to investigate the psychopharmacology of several drugs acting on the dopaminergic systems of the brain (Ljungberg and Ungerstedt, 1978a,b). Though this system probably represents some methodological advance, on a practical level it requires financial resources and computing expertise. More generally, some constraints are still placed on the animal, particularly regarding possible pathways of locomotion and availability of features to receive gnawing, and some behavioural features remain unquantified, e.g. sniffing and rearing. The authors themselves advocate that automated recordings should be complemented by direct visual observation at intervals over each test period.

1.2.3 *Direct visual observation techniques*

It may seem oversimplistic, verging on the naive, to suggest that the best way to investigate the behavioural effects of drugs is to look at each animal and write down what it is seen to be doing over time. However, it does appear that such a simple principle can be developed to define an observational procedure that has advantages over both stereotypy rating scales and automated assessment techniques.

1.2.3.1 *Basic principles.* This means of measuring and analysing the behavioural effects of drugs acting on dopaminergic function has been developed by Fray *et al.* (1980). The basic principle involves defining the presence or absence of differing individual response categories, rather than the occurrence of stereotypy itself, and the major categories of behaviour shown in table 1.4 have been proposed. These authors have found the behavioural categories of swaying (rhythmic swaying movements of the animal's head or body) and grooming to be noted only infrequently, and found it only rarely necessary to resort to a category of miscellaneous behaviour not covered by any of those in Table 1.4. They also advocate that various behaviours should be seen to be performed for minimum time periods, usually at least 3 s, before qualifying for a given category. We will describe below how varying this criterion can influence the results obtained.

Their procedure is as follows: animals who have been habituated to the test cage for periods of 2 h on three previous consecutive days are placed singly in the test cages for a further 30 min habituation period. They are then removed and injected with drug or vehicle and returned to the cage for a 1 h test session. At each 10 min period thereafter, each rat is observed for 10 s by an experimenter unaware of the treatments received by the animals. On each occasion the occurrence of the categories of behaviour given in the table was noted; any combination of these categor-

Table 1.4. Behavioural checklist. (From Fray *et al.* (1980).)

Behavioural category	Description
Still	Asleep or not moving, with an occasional sniff
Locomotion	All four legs moving
Rearing	Both front feet off the cage floor
Sniffing	Sniffing
Licking	Licking
Gnawing	Gnawing
Head down	Animal standing, walking or running with its nose below horizontal

ies could be exhibited by an animal during each single 10 s observation, as they are in no way mutually exclusive. The percentage prevalence of each of these differing response categories can then be determined for the groups of rats receiving the various treatments, at each 10 min interval over the 60 min test period. Varying forms of statistical analysis of such data are described by Fray *et al.* (1980) and in Chapter 7. By utilising such a procedure it was possible to show that apomorphine increased locomotion, sniffing, licking and gnawing but that there were differing dose–response relationships for each of these behaviours. Also, the times of peak exhibition of these various behaviours differed over the test period. These are important data for emphasising that stereotypy ratings by scale do not reflect increasing activation of a unitary process in the brain, and that their use can lead to loss of important information on individual response patterns.

1.2.3.2 *Comparisons with stereotypy rating by scale.* We have adapted this technique and used it in direct comparison with assessment of stereotypy by rating scale, to clarify the relationship between the two procedures. Our technique was as follows.

Animals were habituated to the test cages for a period of 3 h. They were then observed for 1 min for the various categories of behaviour defined by Fray *et al.* (1980), but in addition to noting these individual behavioural categories they were also rated by the stereotypy scale of Creese and Iversen (1973) at the same time. Doses of apomorphine or its vehicle were then administered by an experimenter not involved in the behavioural observations. At 10 min intervals thereafter, this procedure of observation, recording of individual behavioural categories and assessment of stereotypy by rating scale was repeated over a period of 1 h. The percentage of rats exhibiting each behaviour at each time period was then determined.

Using apomorphine doses over the range of 0.125–4.0 mg/kg subcutaneously, sniffing and locomotion were generally potentiated during 10–30 min after drug challenge. Contrary to the finding of Fray *et al.* (1980) we found rearing to be similarly promoted during the same interval. Locomotion and rearing were maximally potentiated by lower doses. Dose–response relationships for promotion of sniffing were influenced by the criterion adopted for allocation of an animal to the sniffing category. If sniffing was defined by the observation of a single episode, however brief and possibly comprising only a single sniff, then 80% of control animals fulfilled this criterion even before apomorphine was given; this obviously left little scope for drug promotion (ceiling effect). If defined by observation of at least a burst of sniffing, as suggested by Fray *et al.*, then 40% of control animals were so categorised at the 20 min point, 100%

being achieved at 0.25 mg/kg (80% at 0.125 mg/kg). Licking was fractionally promoted by 2.0 mg/kg and maximally by 4.0 mg/kg, but only over the later periods of drug action (30–60 min); during earlier periods intense sniffing, with some locomotion and rearing, was seen. Again contrary to the results of Fray and co-workers, we observed very little gnawing behaviour under our conditions. Some of the possible influences of features of the apparatus on response topography will be discussed below.

Regarding the ratings of stereotypy made contemporaneously, peak scores were observed at 20 min after apomorphine challenge for all drug doses except the highest used. Considering stereotypy ratings at the 20 min period, scores increased over 0.125–0.25 mg/kg, with little increase in stereotypy score beyond 0.25 mg/kg; it appeared that ratings indicated a plateau to occur at this dose. The dose-dependent increase in stereotypy score over 0.125–0.25 mg/kg occurs in parallel with the progressive appearance of sniffing, with some locomotion recorded by allocation of individual behavioural categories. The plateau in stereotypy scores thereafter reflects the insensitivity of the scale to the further appearance of rearing and locomotion, which are detected as individual categories over 0.25–2.0 mg/kg. Whereas there is little increase in stereotypy scores over 0.25–4.0 mg/kg at the 20 min point, during the 40–60 min periods licking is prominent with high doses. During these later intervals stereotypy scores superficially appear to show a monotonic increase with dose as they reflect the decline of sniffing to lower doses (0.125–0.5 mg/kg) with drug clearance, the maintenance of sniffing at intermediate doses (1.0–2.0 mg/kg) and the emergence of licking at higher doses (4 mg/kg). Thus this monotonic increase in stereotypy score with apomorphine dose at these later time points may in fact represent an artefactual association of pharmacokinetic factors and the time dependency of response topography, rather than a 'true' dose-response relationship. These effects are illustrated in Fig. 1.3.

1.2.3.3 *Some further refinements of direct visual observation.* In recent studies we have examined the behavioural effects of some novel drugs (Molloy and Waddington, 1984). On the basis of neurochemical studies they have been proposed as dopaminergic agonists with 'selective' actions on certain subtypes of dopamine receptor. We found one drug that produced a non-stereotyped stimulation of behaviour which was difficult to quantify using even the above procedure. The difficulty arose because only certain behaviours were potentiated, principally sniffing and grooming, and even these promoted behaviours did not occur in a true stereotyped fashion, i.e. they were not characterised by invariance, repetition and inappropriateness. Rather, they were potentiated in a dis-

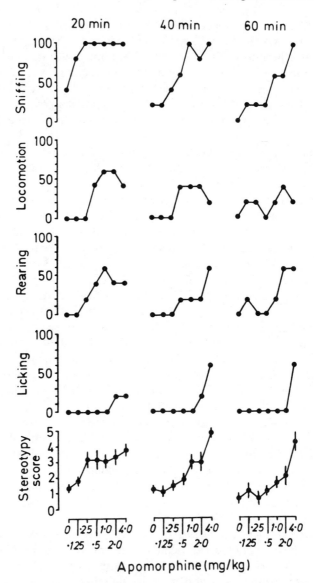

Fig. 1.3.   Incidence of sniffing, locomotion, rearing, and licking behaviours induced by 0.125–4.0 mg/kg apomorphine given subcutaneously into the flank. Data
are expressed as the percentage of individuals in each group showing each behaviour, at 20, 40 and 60 min after challenge with apomorphine. The behavioural
checklist of Table 1.4 was used. Contemporaneous measures of stereotypy were
made using the rating scale indicated in Table 1.3.

continuous, fragmented manner, occurring in short bursts interspersed with periods of quiescence and/or normal activities.

The spectrum of behaviour was completely inappropriate for analysis by rating scale. Even with the above direct visual observation technique, the use of standard observation periods at 10 min intervals provided a usually unrepresentative sample of the behaviours emitted. The discontinuous and fragmented bursts of behaviours seen in preliminary studies seemed to require observations of much shorter duration and of greater frequency. Therefore the following procedure was arrived at. Following habituation, observations were begun at 5 min after drug challenge. Each animal was observed for 5 s in turn (10 animals in total), and all the behaviours seen in that short period were recorded using the list described previously. This was then repeated at 1 min after beginning the first observation and again at 2, 3 and 4 min thereafter. On completion of this sequence the animals were again observed in turn for 5 s each and rated according to the previously described stereotypy scale. This entire 6 min sequence was then repeated after an interval of 4 min (i.e. 10 min after beginning the first observation on the first animal) and continued over a period of 65 min. Thus for each animal this procedure of rapid time sampling generates, at 10 min intervals, five short samples of behaviour over a period of 5 min. It is particularly suited for the assessment of behaviours that are emitted discontinuously, in episodic bursts, and can extract the selective potentiation of one behaviour from several that may be routinely emitted in a non-stereotyped manner.

One more general refinement of direct visual observation techniques has been advocated by Wilcox *et al.* (1979). They describe the use of videotaping of drug effects, with particular reference to stereotypy-inducing agents. It is claimed that analysis of permanent videotape records allows comparisons of differing rating scales and observation techniques under identical 'blind' experimental procedures. A second advantage may reside in their use in training observers and raters to achieve high degrees of efficiency and inter-observer reliability.

There has been much recent interest in refining direct visual observation techniques by way of contemporaneous stereotypy ratings with rapid time-sampling procedures (Molloy and Waddington, 1985), the use of sophisticated movement notation (Szechtman *et al.*, 1985), and the use of microcomputers (Lewis *et al.*, 1985).

1.2.4 *General problems and technical considerations*
1.2.4.1 *Site and mode of injection.* Ljungberg and Ungerstedt (1977a) have reported that the nature of the behavioural response to apomorphine can be influenced by the method of its administration. They investi-

gated both differing sites for subcutaneous injection (into the flank or the dorsal part of the neck) and differing modes of preparation of the apomorphine solution (fast or slow dissolving, with or without ascorbic acid as antioxidant). Among a wide range of behavioural changes associated with various manipulations of these factors, they particularly describe two forms of behavioural response. G-behaviour, characterised by strong compulsive gnawing on the edges of holes in the cage floor (see above description of the apparatus of Ljungberg and Ungerstedt, 1978a), was preferentially induced when apomorphine was dissolved by heating and injected subcutaneously into the flank. LS-behaviour, characterised by increased locomotion and sniffing with repetitive head and limb movements, was preferentially induced when apomorphine was dissolved by heating and injected subcutaneously into the neck, or dissolved by heating together with a high concentration of ascorbic acid and injected into the flank or the neck. Some of the possible explanations for these effects are considered by the authors (Ljungberg and Ungerstedt, 1977a). They indicate the importance of a consistent preparation and site of apomorphine injection, and the necessity to state the conditions used in a given study to allow valid comparisons with the work of others. It is generally agreed that subcutaneous administration of apomorphine is the preferred route, intraperitoneal and oral administration being less effective (Melzacka *et al.*, 1979; Smith *et al.*, 1979). The pharmacokinetics of apomorphine given subcutaneously into the neck and into the flank have not yet been systematically compared. In the studies of Fray *et al.* (1980) described above, apomorphine was given subcutaneously into the neck using 1 mg/ml ascorbic acid as antioxidant; in our own studies we have routinely given subcutaneous injections into the flank, using 1 mg/ml sodium metabisulphite as antioxidant.

Riffee *et al.* (1979) have reported that responsivity to dopamine agonist drugs can be influenced not only by the site of injection but also by pre-injection routines. They have found that pre-administration of vehicle to all animals 1 h before the injection of control and treatment groups with vehicle (again) or apomorphine, respectively, can maximise differences in response between groups and minimise statistical variance. The psychological and/or pharmacological bases of these effects are not known.

1.2.4.2 *Influence of apparatus on qualitative features of response.* Some influences of features of the test apparatus employed on the qualitative nature of responsivity to apomorphine have been investigated by Ljungberg and Ungerstedt (1977b) in their apparatus described previously. When places suitable for gnawing were obscured, much less compulsive gnawing was induced; rather, licking was increased instead, together with some other features of stereotypy. Apomorphine-induced locomotion, however, was not changed when gnawing was restricted. In the preceding comparisons between the work of Fray *et al.* (1980) and ourselves, it is interesting that both studies reported similar data for sniffing and locomotion but not for rearing, gnawing and licking. Our apparatus did not have the wire grid floor or vertical wire sides to provide the opportunities for gnawing present in the apparatus of Fray and co-workers. Therefore their report of gnawing and ours of licking to high apomorphine doses could be accounted for by differing features of the observation cage used. Our cage had an opaque plastic floor (covered with peat moss) and sides, with a metal grid top. This may have favoured the manifestation of rearing. Interestingly, placing the inverted wire grid top of a small mouse cage into the large observation cage (59 cm × 38.5 cm), to provide a surface suitable for gnawing, did not increase the occurrence of this behaviour; licking was still predominantly induced.

In the studies of Ljungberg and Ungerstedt (1977b), some animals were enclosed in a small corner area of the apparatus, to investigate if gnawing behaviour would change when the opportunity for locomotion was restricted. Animals so restricted did in fact gnaw markedly less than those unrestricted. They appeared to attempt vigorously to locomote in the extreme peripheral part of the small enclosed area, away from the features of the area suitable for gnawing. This pattern of locomotion is consistent with that observed in other studies, where stereotyped, perseverative running along a cage wall has been reported after administration of dopaminergic drugs (Schiorring, 1979; Waddington *et al.*, 1982). It would seem necessary in experimental reports to state clearly the features of the apparatus used.

1.2.4.3 *Influence of habituation to apparatus on qualitative features of response.* Several studies have indicated that the extent of the animal's familiarity with the observation cage can have important influences on the form of the behavioural response to dopaminergic drugs. Ljungberg and Ungerstedt (1977b) found that locomotor responses to apomorphine did not differ between animals who were not familiar with (i.e. novel environment) and animals familiar with (i.e. habituated to) the test apparatus. However, gnawing was much less common in animals not familiar with the cage when compared with those who were habituated to the apparatus. Similarly, Mumford *et al.* (1979) have reported that some of the stimulant actions of amphetamine in rats can be obscured by high baseline levels of activity associated with placement in a novel as opposed to a familiar or habituated environment. This is in agreement with the study of Riffee *et al.* (1979), who reported similar results in mice with amphetamine. Interestingly, they found much less consistent effects on responsivity to apomorphine, but it must be noted that electronic activity monitoring, rather than direct visual observation, was utilised.

Just as habituation to the apparatus can influence responsivity to dopaminergic drugs, so manipulations of dopaminergic function can themselves influence the processes of habituation to a novel environment. We have reported that enhancement of dopaminergic function resulting from withdrawal from long-term neuroleptic treatment can attenuate the rate of such habituation effects (Waddington and Gamble, 1980a). In this situation, a 30 min recording of activity, using electronic monitoring, suggested raised activity over this period as a whole. When this 30 min period was resolved into the activity occurring in six successive epochs of 5 min each, levels were initially indistinguishable between control and neuroleptic-withdrawn groups; however, activity was subsequently maintained in the treated animals but showed habituation in controls. When measures obtained over long periods of time are pooled, such temporal information on the distribution of behaviour is lost. Such data may in fact be important indicators of particular drug actions.

1.2.4.4 *Influence of repeated testing of animals with the same drug.* It is tempting to use animals on more than one occasion, with a 'washout' period of variable length being imposed between test sessions to allow clearance of the drug and 'recovery' of the animal. For this to be a valid procedure, it must be clear that the first treatment does not influence the response to the second treatment. Unfortunately, there are several reports indicating that an initial exposure to a dopaminergic drug can indeed influence the response to a second challenge with the same drug or with a different drug.

Ljungberg (1979) has reported on the 'priming' effect of a first apomorphine injection. Such a treatment can importantly influence the qualitative and quantitative features of a second apomorphine challenge given 1–8 h after the first. This first 'priming' injection of apomorphine also influenced spontaneous behaviour in the habituation period immediately preceding the second challenge, over the same inter-trial intervals (1–8 h). The 'priming' effect was seen with doses of apomorphine (0.1 mg/kg subcutaneously) too low to activate animals. Therefore it is not necessary for the animal to be behaviourally stimulated for this effect to occur. No effects were observed with an inter-trial interval of 24 h.

Similar phenomena were investigated by Cools *et al.* (1977), and their results were in some disagreement with those of Ljungberg (1979). However, many methodological factors distinguished these two studies. Cools and co-workers only observed animals between 10 and 20 min. after apomorphine challenge, using non-habituated rats in an apparatus with few surfaces apparently suitable for gnawing. This further attests to the important influences of methodological and procedural variables on the responses observed.

In our own studies, using 0.15 mg/kg of apomorphine given subcutaneously into the flank, we have reported no alteration in stereotyped sniffing when rats were given a second drug challenge 12 days after initial testing (Waddington and Gamble, 1980b). Behaviour was assessed by rating scale, and the results reflected fixated sniffing only. Locomotion, rearing, gnawing and licking were not systematically evaluated over a range of apomorphine doses.

1.2.4.5 *Some other methodological issues.* The data of Ljungberg and Ungerstedt (1977a) and Fray *et al.* (1980) and our own data reported here clearly indicate that the individual behaviours induced by apomorphine have differing time courses following drug challenge. Therefore if, as is common, animals are observed only at a single fixed time after apomorphine challenge, important experimental data may be lost. Time sampling is necessary to overcome this problem. The exact temporal details selected will be influenced by the nature of the behavioural response observed and the duration of action of the drug being investigated, as determined in preliminary studies. In comparing responses to subcutaneous apomorphine in control animals and those withdrawn from long-term neuroleptic treatment, we noted no difference between groups at 10–20 min after challenge, but significant effects were recorded at later times thereafter (Waddington and Gamble, 1980b; Waddington *et al.*, 1981). Therefore, results obtained only at a fixed time after drug challenge may not be truly representative of all the actions of the drug(s) and procedure(s) under investigation.

Recent studies have suggested a circadian rhythm of apomorphine-induced stereotyped behaviour in rats that appears independent of changes in cerebral apomorphine concentrations (Nagayama *et al.*, 1978; Nakano *et al.*, 1980). Using ratings of stereotypy, responsivity to 3 mg/kg of apomorphine given intraperitoneally showed a peak at 17.00 and a trough at 05.00 (Nakano *et al.*, 1980). It is not known if there are distinct circadian influences on the individual components of responsivity to apomorphine. Such data suggest that within a given study, all animals should be tested over the same part of the day; we ourselves routinely make our behavioural observations over 14.00–16.30 only. Circadian effects may be another factor contributing to the differences in results obtained in different laboratories. It is important to note that there appear also to be circadian changes in the behavioural effects of neuroleptics, in terms of their actions on spontaneous behaviour and in antagonising the actions of apomorphine (Nagayama *et al.*, 1978; Campbell and Baldessarini, 1982).

Many of the methodological issues considered here are analysed with regard to behavioural responsivity to apomorphine in the rat. This simply arises from the very widespread use of apomorphine in this species as a prototype dopaminergic agonist. The principles discussed will apply to many other dopaminergic drugs or animal species, though the actual nature of the influence of procedural factors on the behavioural responses they induce may, of course, differ. As a consequence of this, it will be necessary for the experimenter to remain flexible so that procedures can be readily modified to accommodate new behaviours or modes of common, general behaviours that may be observed. An example of this has been given earlier as a refinement of direct visual observation of animals treated with a novel dopaminergic agonist.

It has not been possible to include other behavioural models used in the assessment of dopaminergic function. They are similarly influenced by methodological factors, though they have been less systematically investigated than has stereotyped behaviour. Regarding the turning (rotating/circling) rat model, the methodological problems recognised by Glick *et al.* (1976) have been systematically studied (Waddington and Crow, 1978, 1979a; Waddington, 1979, 1981; Pycock, 1980). Similarly, catalepsy associated with dopamine receptor antagonists has been shown to be markedly influenced by the manner in which it is assessed (Brown and Handley, 1980; Sanberg *et al.*, 1980; de Sousa Moreira *et al.*, 1982).

Whereas the behavioural changes in rodents considered here may appear to be more difficult to quantify objectively than other biological events, it should be recognised that problems can become even more pronounced with the phylogeny of the species studied. In the following chapters, methodological problems in the assessment of non-human primates and man will be similarly considered. It will become apparent that as the range, complexity and subtlety of behaviour increases, so the methodological difficulties associated with their assessment become more prominent.

Acknowledgement

Parts of this work were supported by the Medical Research Council of Ireland and the Royal College of Surgeons in Ireland; the remainder was carried out in the Division of Psychiatry, MRC Clinical Research Centre, Harrow, UK.

References

Baumgarten, H.G., Lachenmayer, L. and Bjorklund, A. (1977). Chemical lesioning of indoleamine pathways. In *Methods in Psychobiology* (R.D. Myers, Ed.), 47–98, Academic Press, New York.
Ben-Ari, Y., Trembley, E., Ottersen, O.P. and Naquet, R. (1979). Evidence suggesting secondary epileptogenic lesions after kainic acid: pretreatment with

diazepam reduces distant but not local damage. *Brain Res.* **165**, 362–5.

Breese, G.R. and Cooper, B.R. (1977). Chemical lesioning: catecholamine pathways. In *Methods in Psychobiology* (R.D. Myers, Ed.), 27–46, Academic Press, New York.

Brown, J. and Handley, S.L. (1980). The development of catalepsy in drug-free mice on repeated testing. *Neuropharmacol.* **19**, 675–8.

Campbell, A. and Baldessarini, R.J. (1982). Circadian changes in behavioural effects of haloperidol in rats. *Psychopharmacol.* **77**, 150–5.

Cools, A.R., Broekkamp, C.L.E. and Van Rossum, J.M. (1977). Subcutaneous injections of apomorphine, stimulus generalisation and conditioning: serious pitfalls for the examiner using apomorphine as a tool. *Pharmacol. Biochem. Behav.* **6**, 705–8.

Costall, B., Naylor, R.J. and Olley, J.E. (1972). The substantia nigra and stereotyped behaviour. *Eur. J. Pharmacol.* **18**, 95–106.

Creese, I. and Iversen, S.D. (1973). Blockage of amphetamine-induced motor stimulation and stereotypy in the adult rat following neonatal treatment with 6-hydroxydopamine. *Brain Res.* **55**, 369–82.

Cross, A.J. and Waddington, J.L. (1981). Striatal kainic acid lesions dissociate ^{3}H-spiperone and ^{3}H-*cis*-flupenthixol binding sites in rat striatum. *Eur. J. Pharmacol.* **71**, 327–32.

de Sousa Moreira, L.F., Pinheiro, M.C. C. and Masur, J. (1982). Catatonic behaviour induced by haloperidol, increased by retesting and elicited without drugs in rats. *Pharmacol.* **25**, 1–5.

Fray, P.J., Sahakian, B.J., Robbins, T.W., Koob, G.F. and Iversen, S.D. (1980). An observational method for quantifying the behavioural effects of dopamine agonists: contrasting effects of d-amphetamine and apomorphine. *Psychopharmacol.* **69**, 253–9.

Gaddy, J.R., Britt, M.D., Neill, D.B. and Haigler, H.J. (1979). Susceptibility of rat neostriatum to damage by kainic acid: age dependence. *Brain Res.* **176**, 192–6.

Gamble, S.J. and Waddington, J.L. (1981). Six months phenothiazine treatment differentially influences distinct dopamine-mediated behaviours. *Brit. J. Pharmacol.* **73**, 240P.

Glick, S.D., Jerussi, T.P. and Fleisher, L.N. (1976). Turning in circles: the neuropharmacology of rotation. *Life Sci.* **18**, 889–96.

Iversen, S.D. and Iversen, L.L. (1981). *Behavioural Pharmacology* (2nd Edn), Oxford University Press, Oxford.

James, T.A. and Starr, M.S. (1978). Effects of the rate and volume of injection on the pharmacological response elicited by intranigral microapplication of drugs in the rat. *J. Pharmacol. Meth.* **1**, 197–200.

Lewis, M.H., Baumeister, A.A., McCorkle, D.L. and Mailman, R.B. (1985). A computerized method for analyzing behavioural observations: studies with stereotypy. *Psychopharmacol.* **85**, 204–9.

Ljungberg, T. (1978). Reliability of two activity boxes commonly used to assess drug induced behavioural changes. *Pharmacol. Biochem. Behav.* **8**, 191–5.

Ljungberg, T. (1979). Evidence that time-related changes in apomorphine stimulation determine the behavioural response. *Neuropharmacol.* **18**, 327–34.

Ljungberg, T. and Ungerstedt, U. (1977a). Different behavioural patterns induced by apomorphine: evidence that the method of administration determines the behavioural response to the drug. *Eur. J. Pharmacol.* **46**, 41–50.

Ljungberg, T. and Ungerstedt, U. (1977b). Apomorphine-induced locomotion and gnawing: evidence that the experimental design greatly influences gnawing while locomotion remains unchanged. *Eur. J. Pharmacol.* **46**, 147–53.

Ljungberg, T. and Ungerstedt, U. (1978a). A method for simultaneous registration of 8 behavioural parameters related to monoamine neurotransmission. *Pharmacol. Biochem. Behav.* **8**, 483–9.

Ljungberg, T. and Ungerstedt, U. (1978b). Classification of neuroleptic drugs according to their ability to inhibit apomorphine-induced locomotion and gnawing: evidence for two different mechanisms of action. *Psychopharmacol.* **56**, 239–47.

McGeer, E.G., Olney, J. and McGeer, P.L. (1978). *Kainic Acid as a Tool in Neurobiology*, Raven Press, New York.

Melzacka, M., Wiszniowska, G., Daniel, W. and Vetulani, J. (1979). Behavioural effects and cerebral pharmacokinetics of apomorphine in the rat: dependence upon the route of administration. *Pol. J. Pharmacol. Pharm.* **31**, 309–17.

Molloy, A.G. and Waddington, J.L. (1984). Dopaminergic behaviour stereospecifically promoted by the D-1 agonist R-SK&F 38393 and selectively blocked by the D-1 antagonist SCH 23390. *Psychopharmacol.* **82**, 409–10.

Molloy, A.G. and Waddington, J.L. (1985). Sniffing, rearing and locomotor responses to the D-1 dopamine agonist R-SK&F 38393 and to apomorphine: differential interactions with the selective D-1 and D-2 antagonists SCH 23390 and metoclopramide. *Eur. J. Pharmacol.* **108**, 305–8.

Mumford, L., Teixeira, A.R. and Kumar, R. (1979). Sources of variation in locomotor activity and stereotypy in rats treated with d-amphetamine. *Psychopharmacol.* **62**, 241–5.

Myers, R.D. (1971). Methods for chemical stimulation of the brain. In *Methods in Psychobiology*, Vol. 1 (R.D. Myers, Ed.), 247–280, Academic Press, London.

Myers, R.D. (1974). *Handbook of Drug and Chemical Stimulation of the Brain*, Van Nostrand Reinhold, New York.

Myers, R.D. and Hoch, D.B. (1978). ^{14}C-Dopamine microinjected into the brainstem of the rat: dispersion kinetics, site content and functional dose. *Brain Res. Bull.* **3**, 601–9.

Nagayama, H., Takagi, A., Nakamura, E. and Yoshida, H. (1978). Circadian susceptibility rhythm to apomorphine in the brain. *Commun. Psychopharmacol.* **2**, 301–10.

Nakano, S., Hara, C. and Ogawa, N. (1980). Circadian rhythm of apomorphine-induced stereotypy in rats. *Pharmacol. Biochem. Behav.* **12**, 459–61.

Olpe, H.R. (1978). Pharmacological manipulations of the automatically recorded biting behaviour evoked in rats by apomorphine. *Eur. J. Pharmacol.* **51**, 441–8.

Pellegrino, L.J. and Cushman, A.J. (1971). Use of stereotaxic technique. In *Methods in Psychobiology*, Vol. 1 (R.D. Myers, Ed.), 67–90, Academic Press, London.

Pycock, C.J. (1980). Turning behaviour in animals. *Neurosci.* **5**, 461–514.

Redgrave, P., Dean, P. and Lewis, G. (1982). A quantitative analysis of stereotyped gnawing induced by apomorphine. *Pharmacol. Biochem. Behav.* **17**, 873–6.

Riffee, W.H., Wilcox, R.E. and Smith, R.V. (1979). Modification of drug-induced behavioural arousal by pre-injection routines in mice. *Psychopharmacol.* **63**, 1–5.

Robbins, T.W. (1977). A critique of the methods available for the measurement of spontaneous motor activity. In *Handbook of Psychopharmacology*, Vol. 7 (L.L. Iversen, S.D. Iversen and S.H. Snyder, Eds), 37–82, Plenum Press, New York.

Robbins, T.W. and Sahakian, B.J. (1981). Behavioural and neurochemical determinants of drug-induced stereotypy. In *Metabolic Disorders of the Nervous
System* (F.C. Rose, Ed.), 244–91, Pitman, London.

Sanberg, P., Pisa, M. and McGeer, E.G. (1979). Strain differences in kainic acid
neurotoxicity. *Brain Res.* **166**,431–5.

Sanberg, P., Pisa, M., Faulks, I.J. and Fibiger, H.C. (1980). Experimental influences on catalepsy. *Psychopharmacol.* **69**, 225–6.

Schiorring, E. (1979). An open field study of stereotyped locomotor activity in
amphetamine-treated rats. *Psychopharmacol.* **66**, 281–7.

Schwarcz, R., Hokfelt, T., Fuxe, K., Jansson, G., Goldstein, M. and Terenius, L.
(1979). Ibotenic acid-induced neuronal degeneration: a morphological and
neurochemical study. *Exp. Brain Res.* **37**, 199–216.

Smith, R.V., Wilcox, R.E., Soine, W.H., Riffee, W.H., Baldessarini, R.J. and
Kula, N.S. (1979). Plasma levels of apomorphine following intravenous, intra-
peritoneal and oral administration to mice and rats. *Res. Commun. Chem.
Pathol. Pharmacol.* **24**, 483–99.

Szechtman, H., Ornstein, K., Teitelbaum, P. and Gonali, I. (1985). The mor-
phogenesis of stereotyped behaviour induced by the dopamine receptor agonist
apomorphine in the laboratory rat. *Neuroscience*, **14**, 783–98.

Tyler, T.D. and Tessel, R.E. (1979). A new device for the simultaneous measurement of locomotor and stereotypic frequency in mice. *Psychopharmacol.* **64**,
285–90.

Waddington, J.L. (1978). Behavioural evidence for GABAergic activity of the
benzodiazepine flurazepam. *Eur. J. Pharmacol.* **51**, 417–22.

Waddington, J.L. (1979). A methodological weakness in the use of neuroleptic
antagonism as a sole criterion for DAergic mediation of drug-induced behavioural effects. *Eur. J. Pharmacol.* **58**, 327–9.

Waddington, J.L. (1980). Effects of nomifensine and desipramine on the sequelae
of intracerebrally-injected 6-OHDA and 5,6-DHT. *Pharmacol. Biochem. Behav.* **13**, 915–17.

Waddington, J.L. (1981). Relationship between functional supersensitivity and
extent of denervation of dopamine receptors. *Physiol. Behav.* **26**, 627–9.

Waddington, J.L. and Cross, A.J. (1978). Neurochemical changes following
kainic acid lesions of the nucleus accumbens. *Life Sci.* **22**, 1011–14.

Waddington, J.L. and Crow, T.J. (1978). Methodological problems in the
measurement of drug-induced rotational behaviour. *Psychopharmacol.* **58**, 153–
5.

Waddington, J.L. and Crow, T.J. (1979a). Rotational responses to serotonergic
and dopaminergic agonists after unilateral dihydroxytryptamine lesions of the
medial forebrain bundle. *Life Sci.* **25**, 1307–14.

Waddington, J.L. and Crow, T.J. (1979b). Drug-induced rotational behaviour
following unilateral intracerebral injection of saline/ascorbate solution. *Brain
Res.* **161**, 371–6.

Waddington, J.L. and Gamble, S.J. (1980a). Neuroleptic treatment for a substantial period of adult life: behavioural sequelae of 9 months haloperidol administration. *Eur. J. Pharmacol.* **67**, 363–9.

Waddington, J.L. and Gamble, S.J. (1980b). Spontaneous activity and apomorphine stereotypy during and after withdrawal from 3½ months continuous
administration of haloperidol: some methodological issues. *Psychopharmacol.*
71, 75–7.

Waddington, J.L. and Longden, A. (1977). Rotational behaviour and cGMP
responses following manipulations of nigral mechanisms with chlordiazepoxide.

Naunyn-Schmiedeberg's Arch. Pharmacol. **300**, 233–7.

Waddington, J.L., Gamble, S.J. and Bourne, R.C. (1981). Sequelae of 6 months continuous administration of *cis*(Z)- and *trans*(E)-flupenthixol in the rat. *Eur. J. Pharmacol.* **69**, 511–13.

Waddington, J.L., Cross, A.J., Gamble, S.J. and Bourne, R.C. (1982). Functional heterogeneity of multiple dopamine receptors during 6 months treatment with distinct classes of neuroleptic drugs? In Advances in Dopamine Research (M. Kohsaka, Ed.), 143–6, Pergamon Press, Oxford.

Wilcox, R.E., Riffee, W.H. and Smith, R.V. (1979). Videotaping: the evaluation of stereotypic effects of antiparkinsonian agents. *Pharmacol. Biochem. Behav.* **10**, 161–4.

Wolf, G. (1971). Elementary histology for neuropsychologists. In *Methods in Psychobiology*, Vol. 1 (R.D. Myers, Ed.), 281–300, Academic Press, London.

Wolfarth, S., Coelle, E.-R., Osborne, N.N. and Sontag, K.-H. (1977). Evidence for a neurotoxic effect of ascorbic acid after an intranigral injection in the cat. *Neurosci. Lett.* **6**, 183–6.

Wuerthele, S.M., Lovell, K.L., Jones, M.Z. and Moore, K.E. (1978). A histological study of kainic acid-induced lesions in the rat brain. *Brain Res.* **149**, 487–97.

Use of the Common Marmoset (*Callithrix jacchus*) in Psychopharmacological Research

2.1 Introduction, housing and maintenance

Old World monkeys, of which the rhesus monkey (*Macaca mulatta*) is the most familiar, have been used for many years in the study of primate learning ability and cognitive function, and much has been learnt of the social lives of these animals. Most of the work has been carried out with a view to understanding the mechanisms underlying the sub-human primate's capabilities, and has until comparatively recently been the province of the ethologist and the animal psychologist (e.g. Köhler, 1925; Harlow, 1949). More recently, with the emergence of psychopharmacology and biological psychiatry as distinct components of neuroscience, the extensive behavioural repertoire of the sub-human primates has become increasingly exploited as attempts have been made to investigate the possibilities of modelling both neurological and psychiatric conditions. For example the role of the temporal lobes in learning and memory and the sequelae of accidental damage to temporal lobe structures are being extensively investigated in primates with surgical ablations of these structures, and a wealth of information concerning the origins of amnesia in humans has been derived from these experiments (Mishkin *et al.*, 1982). Similarly many researchers have attempted to set up models of the most common psychiatric conditions, from the pioneering work of Harlow on the effects of early separation and social deprivation to more recent attempts at producing analogues of the symptoms of schizophrenia by treating monkeys with drugs that are psychotogenic in humans (see Harlow, 1962; Randrup and Munkvad, 1967; Ellison *et al.*, 1981). Old World monkeys have also been used to study the metabolic effects of psychoactive drugs; however, since these animals are expensive to purchase and maintain, terminal experiments are not frequently undertaken and techniques have had to be developed in order to sample body fluids (see Baker and Ridley, 1979; Joseph *et al.*, 1981).

Increasing difficulty and expense in obtaining, keeping and breeding Old World monkeys has led to the growing use of small New World monkeys for behavioural and physiological research. The genus *Callithrix*, of which the common marmoset (*C. jacchus*) is the most numerous member, comprises probably the simplest phylogenetically, and is among the smallest of the true primates. Common marmosets have a predominantly grey–brown body with large white tufts over the ears and a grey–brown ringed tail. They live in the tops of the trees in the tropical forests of the Amazon basin, feeding on fruit, vegetable matter and insects. The marmoset has proved to be most useful as an experimental animal since it is hardy, breeds well in captivity and presents no exceptional hazards when compared with other larger monkeys.

Common marmosets live in stable family groups with sophisticated parental care and rapid reproductive frequency which, together with its small size, makes this species particularly useful for the study of development and social interaction. In captivity animals live for 10–12 years, becoming sexually mature at 12–18 months. Gestation time is about 140 days with mating resuming from one week post partum. The diagnosis of pregnancy in the marmoset can be difficult in the early stages although kits have been developed for the qualitative estimation of chorionic gonadotrophin in this species (Hodgen *et al.*, 1976). Many workers, however, believe that abdominal palpation is at least as reliable a method for detecting pregnancy after about 11–20 days (Phillips and Grist, 1975; Lunn *et al.*, 1979).

Marmosets usually produce twins which, though not monozygotic, are uniplacental, and have proved useful in our laboratory in matched-pair experimental designs. It is said that the male will assist the female during delivery, which usually takes place at night. After the placenta is expelled it is eaten by the parents and other members of the family. From birth the male carries the infants for much of the time, returning them to the female for feeding and, within a few days, older siblings can also be seen carrying them. The frequent production of triplets is a complication, often associated with birth difficulties, when one infant may be stillborn. When three live infants are born, one or two may die from inadequate nutrition although this may be overcome by supplementary feeding or hand-rearing. Hearn and Burden (1979) have described a method in which each infant is removed from the mother for 12 h in rotation and hand-fed during that time, although Ziegler *et al.* (1981) suggest that the least time consuming and most successful method is to leave all three infants with their mother but to give two supplementary feeds to each infant per day. Occasionally, if there happens to be another lactating female with only one infant, a triplet can be successfully cross-fostered. This can best be achieved by removing the singleton from the mother and putting it with the triplet to be fostered in a warm place until they have acquired each other's smell. They can then be returned to the foster mother. Despite these efforts a high infant mortality is to be expected (Poole and Evans, 1982). Looking at 13 females selected as good breeders over a five-year period we found a 20% perinatal mortality with further deaths during the first year such that only about 60% of offspring reached maturity. Thus although females may have two pregnancies per year, the overall production may only be two surviving infants per female-year.

In our laboratory, marmosets are kept in a large colony room maintained at 20–25°C with a relative humidity of 50% and a 12-h light/dark cycle. Ideally, each family group, which may consist of two adults, two adolescents and two infants, should be housed in a cage which is not less than 1 m^3 (Ingram, 1975), although for ethological studies much larger structures have been employed (Stevenson and Poole, 1976). Single animals kept for experimental purposes may be housed in smaller cages (e.g. 30 cm × 50 cm × 50 cm) fitted with a dark nestbox in which the animals can sleep and with wooden perches which they can use for scent-marking and gnawing. These cages should be cleaned regularly. If they are allowed to become dirty, the condition of the marmosets will deteriorate and their coats will become greasy and matted. Although marmosets tolerate caging better than other primates, animals kept individually in small cages will develop cage stereotypies consisting of repetitive locomotor sequences, particularly somersaulting around the cage. They do not, however, develop the severely disturbed and self-injurious behaviour seen in some caged primates even if they are reared in isolation. For discussion of stereotypies see Ridley and Baker (1982, 1983). Infants are best left with their parents for 12–18 months after which they can be removed from their home cages and placed with suitable mates. When adults have been established in pairs for some time without producing offspring, they can be re-paired, sometimes with fruitful results. When animals are introduced to each other for the first time, it is important to watch them closely until they get used to each other. Occasionally, bouts of aggression will occur which might prove damaging or even fatal for one of them. Gangs of adolescent males can be kept successfully but females are more temperamental. Keeping mixed-sex gangs usually ends in trouble.

To meet the marmoset's daily dietary requirement a convenient selection can be made from a variety of fruits, bread, egg and monkey chow supplemented weekly with bone-marrow extract, although care must be taken to ensure that the diet is well balanced. A condition of poor weight gain and weakness termed 'marmoset wasting syndrome' has been found which may be associated with overfeeding (as well as underfeeding) where the animal may choose the less nutritious but more palatable dietary items such as fruit rather than the more nutritious monkey pellets. Shimwell *et al.* (1979) recommend that a high protein intake be maintained especially during the weaning period in order to avoid the development of this condition. A supplement of vitamin D_3 and calcium is essential otherwise young animals will develop rickets, and older animals (particularly breeding females) may develop osteoporosis. For a more comprehensive discussion of the maintenance and breeding of the common marmoset (including hand-rearing techniques) the reader is referred to Stevenson (1976) and Poole and Evans (1982).

2.2 Legal requirements and safety precautions

All monkeys imported into the British Isles are required by law to be isolated for six months in an approved quarantine facility. A Home Office licence, which permits the experimenter to use animals, together with the certificates which specify exactly the procedures to be used, are required for most of the procedures described in subsequent sections of this chapter. If primates are used, a special application must also be made.

The safety precautions required when handling simians are discussed in Perkins and O'Donoghue (1969). It is recommended that persons entering the colony should wear protective clothing including gowns, which should be sterilised after use, and disposable gloves, masks, caps and overshoes. This will help to prevent cross-infection (in either direction) and will protect workers from contamination with the particularly pungent urine. Frequent handling of marmosets from birth renders these animals relatively tame and consequently more amenable to injections and other simple procedures. Nevertheless, an adult marmoset is capable of inflicting a painful bite and is occasionally enthusiastic in its attempts, so heavy leather gloves should be worn when handling these animals.

Although the major viral hazards usually connected with simians (virus B, Marburg virus and rabies) have not been specifically associated with New World monkeys, a variety of herpetic viruses have been identified in some New World species. Some of these viruses are known to be oncogenic when transmitted experimentally from the host to other primate species and the possibility of a pathogenic effect in man cannot be ruled out. Unlike some other species of marmosets and tamarins the common marmoset is not susceptible to viral hepatitis.

The most important non-viral disease associated with monkey handling is tuberculosis although common marmosets seem to be resistant to this disease and it is not considered a hazard in this species. These animals are, however, susceptible to a variety of enteric disorders, and occasional bouts of diarrhoea, which may prove fatal in infants, are not uncommon. Simian shigellosis and salmonellosis are not confined to any one primate species, and both shigellae and salmonellae have been isolated from marmosets with enteric disorders. The spread of salmonella to humans has not been reported, but there have been many reported cases of shigellosis in humans which have been attributed to contact with monkeys, so extra care is required when infection is suspected. Every occurrence of diarrhoea should be treated seriously and the animals involved must be administered a kaolin/broad-spectrum antibiotic mixture while the causative organism is being identified. Once the identification and sensitivity are established, a specific antibiotic should be used. It must be recognised, however, that long-term antibiotic treatment can alter the normal balance of gut flora resulting in acute gastric dilatation (Stein *et al.*, 1981). For this reason the use of antibiotics as a prophylactic should not be considered.

As mentioned earlier, barrier clothing is worn to protect the animals as well as the experimenter. Marmosets are known to be experimentally susceptible to herpes simplex (associated with coldsores in humans) which may produce systemic illness with high mortality rates, and to measles virus (Hunt *et al.*, 1978). It is not clear how readily measles virus transmits to marmosets, and reports of the occurrence of the disease in these animals is rare although an outbreak reported by Levy and Mircovic (1971) resulted in the deaths of 326 animals over six months in one colony. In this laboratory a virus infection of the respiratory tract spread rapidly through the marmoset colony eventually affecting about one-half of the animals (35/75) and resulting in the deaths of three (Flecknell *et al.*, 1982). The virus was identified as a para-influenza virus (Sendai virus — associated with rodents), emphasising the need for rigorous attention to personal hygiene and the wearing of clean protective clothing when moving from rodent rooms to the monkey colony. We would suggest further that workers thought to be suffering from upper respiratory tract infections should be discouraged from entering the colony.

Safety precautions over and above those taken in the day-to-day running of a marmoset colony will be necessary if experiments involving known pathogens or materials suspected of being pathogenic are to be conducted in monkeys. Research establishments usually draw up their own regulations governing the handling of simians under such circumstances after reference to the Howie Report (1978).

2.3 General Techniques

2.3.1 *Anaesthesia*
For light anaesthesia or immobilisation, 0.05–0.1 ml 50 mg/ml Ketamine injected into the thigh muscle will suffice. This will produce immobilisation and considerable analgesia within a few minutes, which will last for 10–15 min during which simple procedures can be carried out, e.g. the administration of an intravenous injection. Ketamine is not recommended for painful or operative procedures since the degree of insensibility cannot be assumed from the lack of movement. Saffan (0.8 ml/kg) given intramuscularly is a short-acting anaesthetic suitable for minor operative procedures.

For a more profound anaesthesia lasting 2–3 h suitable for major operative procedures, 0.05 ml 50 mg/ml Ketamine should be followed by 0.15 ml 60 mg/ml sodium pentobarbitone (Nembutal) administered intraperitoneally. The depth of anaesthesia can be estimated from the response to touching the eye or pinching the foot or tail. If required, a supplementary intramuscular injection of 0.05 ml 50 mg/ml Ketamine can be given after 2 h. Marmosets tolerate anaesthesia well but after an anaesthetic the animal should not be returned to a shared cage until it has regained consciousness. An unconscious or semi-conscious animal could be mutilated by other animals. If a particularly rapid or deep anaesthesia is required for a terminal procedure (e.g. perfusion), 0.15 ml 60 mg/ml sodium pentobarbitone may be injected directly into the right lung using a 25 g needle. Following Ketamine immobilisation the animal is held on its back and the needle is inserted between the ribs just below the nipple. No terminal procedure should be commenced until the animal is deeply anaesthetised.

2.3.2 *Methods of drug administration*

Oral administration of an approximate dosage of drugs can be achieved by adding the drug to a limited water supply. Marmosets like sweet foods, and the unpleasant or bitter taste of some drugs can be masked by the addition of blackcurrant-flavoured cordial to the water. Suspension of drugs in fruit-flavoured syrup (usually prepared for paediatric use) can be administered to a hand-held animal by using a 1 ml syringe without a needle. These methods are particularly suitable for the administration of antibiotics.

Intramuscular injections of 0.1–0.2 ml can be achieved using a 25 g needle while holding the animal in the heavily gloved left hand, though this requires practice to be carried out efficiently. The marmoset is held front downwards in the palm of the left hand; the tail is held between the third and fourth fingers and the right leg between the second and third fingers. The fur on this leg is wetted with alcohol and parted so that the injection site can be clearly seen. The muscle on the outside of the thigh is a suitable site if care is taken not to push the needle towards the bone (see Fig. 2.1.).

Much larger volumes (up to 0.6–0.7 ml) can be injected by the intraperitoneal route, although two people may be required if it is to be carried out without anaesthetic. This method of injection is likely to be more painful than the intramuscular route, and if the animal jerks during the injection internal injury may result. For this reason we would advise the use of light Ketamine anaesthesia. The animal is laid on its back with arms and legs held down. The lower belly is grasped about the midline between the forefinger and thumb of the left hand and pulled gently upwards. The needle (25 g short) can then be pushed through into the peritoneal cavity about 2 cm to the right of the midline taking care not to puncture either of the two major blood vessels which run down the middle of the abdomen. The site chosen should be low enough to avoid injecting into the liver, which could prove fatal.

Intravenous injections are not easy in the marmoset and are best attempted in the tail under Ketamine anaesthesia. After shaving off the fur, a modest sized vein can be located on either side of the base of the tail which can be punctured using a 27 g needle. Other intravenous methods are not recommended.

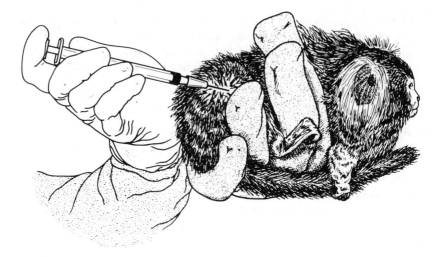

Fig. 2.1. Intramuscular injection technique.

2.3.3 *Sampling of body fluids*

Urine collection presents no problem as there are a large variety of
rodent metabolic cages which can be modified to accommodate a marmoset. Blood can be withdrawn with some difficulty from the femoral
vein under light Ketamine anaesthesia. Up to 100 μl cerebrospinal fluid
(CSF) can be withdrawn by cisternal puncture from a lightly anaesthetised adult animal. The head is held firmly, using the ear bars of a
stereotaxic frame (see below) and the face is pushed downwards as far as
possible. The nape of the neck is shaved and a 26 g short butterfly
needle is inserted to a depth of approximately 4 mm at 90° to the back of
the head on the midline. The tip of the needle may encounter the bone of
the back of the skull and would then have to be manipulated until it is
centred over the membrane covering the cistern. Puncturing this membrane can sometimes be felt as a slight 'give'. Over-insertion often results
in a sharp twitch by the animal, and a slight retraction usually then
produces CSF (see Fig. 2.2).

Withdrawal of CSF should not be forced beyond that which is readily
available. With practice clear samples can be obtained, though pulling on
the syringe too hard may contaminate the sample with blood. Blood-
stained samples should be discarded and puncture reattempted after a
period of several days, although excessive repetition should be avoided.
To date we have attempted about 100 cisternal punctures with more than
90% producing useful CSF samples. The remainder were usually blood
stained and, very occasionally, CSF was unobtainable. Only one animal
has shown noticeable trauma consisting of ataxia and weakness of the

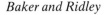

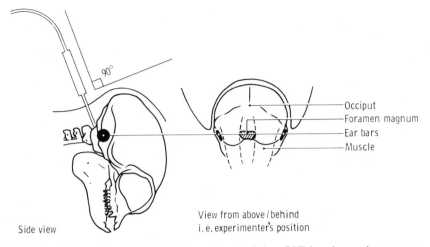

Side view

View from above / behind
i. e. experimenter's position

Occiput
Foramen magnum
Ear bars
Muscle

Fig. 2.2. Illustration of the technique for obtaining CSF by cisternal puncture.

hind legs which lasted for 24 h. Subsequent attempts in this animal were successful. This procedure should be carried out before daily feeding otherwise copious vomiting may occur as the animal recovers from the anaesthetic.

2.4 Stereotaxic techniques

Ideally, surgical procedures using marmosets should be carried out under aseptic conditions though stereotaxic procedures involving single small drill-holes may be successfully carried out under 'clean' conditions.

For the techniques described in this section a standard rat stereotaxic apparatus (e.g. David Kopf Instruments No. 900) fitted with a primate head holder based on David Kopf Instruments No. 945 can be used. The eye pieces should be ground down so that the ends are no bigger than 2 mm in diameter, but should maintain the lower (definitive) position. The mouth piece should be similarly diminished and should protrude 5 mm beyond the eye pieces (see Fig. 2.3).

2.4.1 *Injections*
For stereotaxically positioned injections (e.g. of neurotoxins) into discrete areas of the brain, the syringe should be clamped to the gantry and, after centring the ear bars on the frame, the gantry position should be adjusted till the needle just meets the point where the ear bars touch. The anterior–posterior (AP), lateral (L) and vertical (V) coordinates are then read off the gantry scales and represent the zero coordinates of the

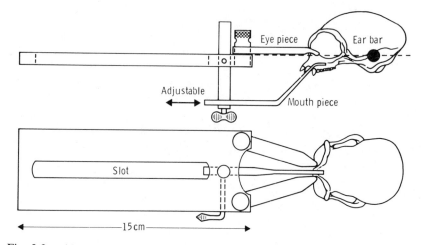

Fig. 2.3. A stereotaxic head holder suitable for a marmoset.

system. Using these readings in conjunction with a standard stereotaxic atlas of the marmoset brain (Stephan *et al.*, 1980), any position in the animal's brain can be specified. Having established the frame zero, the gantry is swung to one side and the anaesthetised animal (with head shaved) is held by the ear bars. The bars are positioned so that the head is located in the centre of the frame. The head is held firmly by locating the eye pieces on the lower rim of the eye sockets and the mouth piece on the roof of the mouth. The eyes may be protected with a drop of liquid paraffin. When the mouth piece is in position, the lower jaw should be pulled down and the tongue allowed to fall forward to prevent choking. If the head is positioned correctly there will be no movement. For a single injection a small longitudinal incision is made to expose the skull. The correct settings for the needle are calculated, and having set the AP and L settings the gantry is swung back to the working position. The needle is lowered on to the skull and the entry point is marked. The gantry is again swung to one side and a small hole is drilled in the skull at the point of entry using a hand drill. The meninges, which are exceedingly tough compared with those of the rat, should be punctured with a 25 g needle prior to insertion of the injection needle. The gantry is then returned to the working position and the needle lowered through the hole in the skull to the correct coordinate position (V), determined from the atlas. In order to minimise tissue damage, injections should be carried out slowly over several minutes and the needle left in position for several more minutes before removal to prevent injected material from rising in the injection tract. When the injection is complete, the needle is lifted, the gantry swung to the rest position and the incision closed. In order to ensure rapid and complete healing and to prevent the animal from pulling out the stitches, either 'subcutaneous' or 'mattress' stitching is recommended using silk sutures (see Fig. 2.4). When healing is complete these stitches can be removed. Autoclips should not be used. If required, a topical antibiotic can be applied and the wound is covered, finally, by plastic skin. For more than one injection the whole of the top of the skull can be exposed by making one skin incision across the head just in front of the ears. The skin can be pulled apart to reveal the complete skull top. For multiple injections or suction lesions a bone flap can be turned. After the skull has been exposed, the temporal muscle is cut on one side of the head. Small drill-holes are made at intervals around the perimeter of the dome of the skull and joined up with a dental saw or fine fret-saw. On easing up this flap, the bone under the remaining temporal muscle cracks and the bone flap can be turned back using this muscle as a hinge. The flap should be kept covered with a saline-soaked swab. This method allows viewing of the surface of the meninges while making stereotaxic injections. Depression of the surface of the brain by the injection needle can be compensated for and meningeal bleeding can be stopped using diathermy. Having completed the injections, the bone is repositioned and the temporal muscle rejoined using fine silk sutures. The skin incision is closed in the usual way. Marmosets tolerate these procedures well, and in

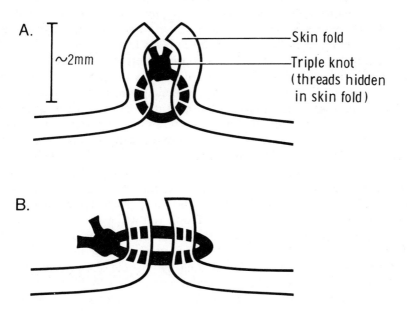

A.
~2mm
Skin fold
Triple knot
(threads hidden
in skin fold)

B.

Fig. 2.4. A, Subcutaneous skin sutures suitable for use in primates; B, an alternative, easier method.

a series of 16 such operations in our laboratory (each involving 10 injections), immediate post-operative mortality was zero. Two animals died
after 10–14 days though their deaths may have been due to the biological
material which was injected.

2.4.2 *Intracerebral in-dwelling cannulae*

Drug injection into specific brain sites in unanaesthetised animals is a
useful method of localising their action. We have found that implanted
cannulae remain patent in the marmoset for about 6 months (and sometimes much longer) before accident or infection take their toll. Prior to
implantation of the cannulae (Clark Electromedical Instruments) the
monkey's head is measured stereotaxically under Ketamine anaesthesia
and the inner and outer cannulae are shortened so that when the end of
the inner cannula is positioned at the required stereotaxic coordinates,
the base of the external part of the outer cannula will be sitting on the
surface of the skull.

Surgery is carried out under Nembutal anaesthesia. The skull is exposed by a large semi-circular incision around the occiput. The inner and
outer cannula assembly is mounted in the stereotaxic frame together with
a section of hypodermic needle fitted over the cannula. A hole is drilled
in the skull at the appropriate point of entry. Two further holes are
drilled around this central hole and fitted with 12 BA short brass screws.
The cannula assembly is lowered until the hypodermic needle has punctured the meninges. The cannula is then withdrawn, the hypodermic
needle is removed and the cannula assembly is lowered again until the tip
of the inner cannula reaches the appropriate stereotaxic position. A small
portion of the skull may have to be drilled away using a dental drill if the
cannula assembly is too short. The exposed area of bone is dried using a
jet of compressed air, and a mound of dental cement is built up around
the cannula and covering the two brass screws (acting as anchor points).
The whole assembly is held in the stereotaxic frame until the dental
cement is quite hard. The inner cannula is then withdrawn leaving the
outer (or guide) cannula in position. As small a hole as possible is made
in the skin to accommodate the outer cannula and the skin incision is
closed. The outer cannula is fitted with a keeper and the animal is then
allowed to recover. The problem of skin retraction over the dental cement is considerably reduced if the stitching is as far away from the
cannula as possible. Post-operative recovery is excellent although animals
are best housed separately for as long as possible since grooming and
picking may introduce infection to the wound. We have employed this
technique to study the effects of bilateral injection of amphetamine into
the caudate and accumbens nuclei using two cannulae in diagonal orientation (see Fig. 2.5).

Intracerebral injections in unanaesthetised animals can be greatly facili-

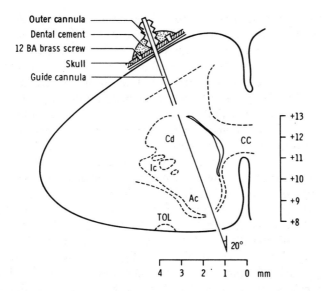

Fig. 2.5. Diagram to illustrate cannula implant. In this example a diagonal orientation traversing the striatum was used. CC: corpus callosum, Cd: caudate, AC: nucleus accumbens, IC: internal capsule and TOL: olfactory tract.

tated if the animals are held firmly in a restraining chair. We have designed a small chair consisting of a sturdy pillar attached to a base which is clamped to a bench. Fixed to the top of the pillar is a flat platform with a central hole through which the animal puts its head. An adjustable collar then fits snugly around the head and markedly restricts movement. The marmoset's body is wrapped in a towel and strapped to the pillar. We have found that our monkeys quickly adapt to this procedure and remain quiet during the injections.

This technique can also be used for intracerebroventricular injections. It has been our experience that such injections can conveniently be made into the trigone of the lateral ventricles such that fluid flows into all three arms of the lateral ventricular system. A coordinate 1 mm below that indicated by the stereotaxic atlas will ensure that the ependyma is punctured and will allow fluid to reflux into the ventricles. Volumes of $5-15$ μl in each hemisphere are suitable, though consideration should be given to the pH and concentration of the drug employed. Such injections can be made without anaesthesia using the primate chair.

2.5 Perfusion and brain dissection

Fixation of brain tissue in formalin for histological examination is greatly improved by exsanguination and perfusion since the size of the brain ($7-8$ g fresh weight, $7-8$ ml volume, $34 \times 20 \times 25$ mm maximum dimensions)

renders fixation by immersion slow. The animal should be *deeply* anaesthetised with Nembutal during this procedure. The thoracic cavity is
opened and the pericardium dissected away as quickly as possible.
Approximately 250 ml of normal saline followed by 250 ml 10% formol-
saline under 1 m head of pressure (i.e. hung from a convenient position)
should be run through a large diameter needle into the left ventricle of
the heart, after a small puncture has been made in the right ventricle.
When the perfusion is complete, the scalp is cut away and the roof of the
skull is removed using bone nibblers, starting at the foramen magnum.
The meninges must be dissected away, especially from around the cerebellum and above the corpus callosum. The head is inverted and the optic
chiasm, cranial nerves and spinal cord are cut so that the brain can be
eased gently out. Fresh brains can be removed by the same procedure
though more care is needed so as not to damage the structure.

Dissection of specific brain areas is most conveniently achieved by
freezing the brain, slicing it into 2–3 mm sections and removing the
required area after reference to the stereotaxic atlas. A rapid, fresh
dissection can be made by cutting through the corpus callosum and peel-
ing back the cortex above the lateral ventricles to reveal the structures
of the basal ganglia underneath.

2.6 Methods of behavioural assessment

2.6.1 *Direct observation*
The general behaviour and social interactions in groups of common
marmosets have been studied extensively using methods of direct
observation, and a complete ethogram of this species has been published
(Stevenson and Poole, 1976). In our studies on the effects of psychotropic
drugs on behaviour, we have found that these monkeys are best observed
through a one-way mirror or smoked perspex window since they tend to
direct a considerable proportion of their behaviour towards a visible
observer. Behaviour can be scored either as occurrences, i.e. the number
of bouts of eating, locomotion, grooming, etc. in a given period of time,
or it can coded every second (or few seconds) over time so that a measure
of the duration of episodes of different categories of behaviour can be
obtained. Either method can be greatly facilitated by the use of a micro-
processor (e.g. the CBM Pet) to accumulate coded data and to perform
subsequent statistical manipulations. The method of coding behaviour
every second over short periods of time has been used in marmosets to
study both acute and chronic effects of drugs on behaviour (Scraggs and
Ridley, 1978; Ridley *et al.*, 1979a). A few sessions of observation are
usually sufficient to ensure reasonable reliability between observers. The
procedure usually adopted in our laboratory consists of observing each

animal for 50 s (i.e. 50×1 s observations) at a time before moving on to the next animal. When all the animals have been rated, the procedure is repeated in the same order. In this way each animal is observed for a total of 100 s and the percentage of time spent on each behaviour can be readily expressed. The frequency with which behavioural observations are made will depend, of course, on the nature of the experiment. In a test of inter-observer reliability, three normal marmosets were assessed for 50 s each by three observers (A, B, C). Inter-observer correlations were r_{AB} = 0.99, r_{AC} = 0.99, r_{BC} = 0.98, and no significant difference between observers was found (X^2 = 4.2, d.f. = 8, see Table 2.1). Behaviour is usually most variable in normal, untreated animals; where treatments induce particular types of behavioural response, inter-observer correlations can be expected to improve.

2.6.1.1 *Behavioural effects of amphetamine and apomorphine and their antagonism.* We have used the methods of quantified direct observation to assess the major behavioural effects of amphetamine and apomorphine in the marmoset and have studied their antagonism by various neuroleptic drugs. Five mutually exclusive categories of behaviour were used in these experiments.

(1) Inactivity: as the name suggests the animals were doing nothing. They were either awake but sitting quite still or were asleep.
(2) Checking: an interesting behaviour characterised by small rapid head movements in the horizontal plane and probably associated with continuous monitoring of the environment. Undrugged marmosets usually spend 15–20% of their time in this category.
(3) Locomotion: all behaviours associated with movement of the whole body were assigned to this category, including slow walking around the cage, running, jumping, etc.

Table 2.1 An example of inter-observer reliability on simple classification of behaviour occurring in one 150-s reading in a group of three marmosets.

Behavioural category	Observer A	Observer B	C	Total
Inactivity	68	71	66	205
Checking	14	10	19	43
Locomotion	15	13	14	42
Contact	41	46	43	130
Activities	12	10	8	30
Total	150	150	150	450

X^2 = 4.2   d.f. = 8 (not significant)

(4) Activities: marmosets spend a great deal of their time manipulating objects with their hands, eating, drinking and self-grooming. All these behaviours were grouped in this category.

(5) Contact: this category consisted of any contact between the animal under observation and others, including huddling together (which these animals like to do) as well as all grooming, sexual activity, playing and fighting.

We found that amphetamine induced a dose-dependent increase in *checking* and a reciprocal decrease in *inactivity* but no change in *locomotion*, over the range 0.5–4.0 mg/kg i.m. with a time course of about 1.5 h for the main effects. This was followed by a gradual return to normal behaviour over the following 4 h (Ridley *et al.*, 1980a). At 4.0 mg/kg amphetamine, animals spent about 80% of their time checking during the first hour after injection. Each animal sat on a perch or hung from the bars of the cage and engaged in small-amplitude, rapid, jerky head movements, which some have described as hypervigilance. Our experiments suggest, however, that this amphetamine-induced *checking* is not visually directed but is internally generated (Ridley *et al.*, 1980a). During this time animals minimised *contact* with one another, usually disposing themselves about the cage so as to maximise the distance between them. At doses greater than 4 mg/kg, severe stereotypy was observed, comprising padding movements of the hands and feet, slow creeping movements and rigid immobility. The *d*-isomer of amphetamine was found to have about twice the potency of the *l*-isomer for *checking*, and both isomers suppressed purposeful *activities* and *contact* over a wide dose range (Scraggs and Ridley, 1978). Amphetamine-induced *checking* was suppressed by pretreating the animals with haloperidol, metoclopramide or muscimol, but was unaffected by propranolol, aceperone, diazepam, sulpiride or baclofen (Scraggs and Ridley, 1979; Ridley *et al.*, 1979b, 1980c). The behavioural response of marmosets to amphetamine is very reliable across animals, whereas in other primates stereotyped behaviour after amphetamine is often complex and idiosyncratic (Randrup and Munkvad, 1967). This lack of variation between animals makes the marmoset a particularly useful primate in which to study drug effects. Studies using intracerebral cannulae suggest that amphetamine injected into the nucleus accumbens has more effect on checking, locomotion and social interaction than amphetamine injected into the caudate nucleus (Annett *et al.*, 1983).

When amphetamine was administered via the drinking water up to a dose of 4 mg/kg/day over a total of 16 weeks (Ridley *et al.*, 1979a), the increase in checking gradually subsided during the first 4 weeks although social contact was not reinstated. The animals began to engage in destructive self-grooming behaviour, however, where each animal would scratch or pick at a focal point on its body, usually forearm, thigh or tail, for long periods of time. Eventually bald patches with sores began to appear and there was a risk of infection. When we considered that the health of the animals was in jeopardy, we added haloperidol to the drinking water (still containing amphetamine). Addition of this neuroleptic to the drug regime produced a transient sedation and abolished self-grooming immediately but did not overcome the loss of social contact. When haloperidol was withdrawn, a rebound increase in checking was seen. Social contact returned promptly in the final phase of the experiment when amphetamine was withdrawn (Ridley *et al.*, 1979a).

When marmosets were treated acutely by i.m. injection with the direct dopamine agonist apomorphine, at doses of less than 1 mg/kg, a biphasic response was observed. Vomiting was common 2-4 min after injection, locomotion and checking were both increased in the first 30 min, but then the animals became quiescent or somnolent for several hours. The effects of 1 mg/kg apomorphine or higher were dramatically different from those of the lower doses. Because the behavioural categories used hitherto were inappropriate, and as the drug effects seemed to be life threatening, we confined our observations to just four animals. No vomiting was seen at this dose in any of the animals. Almost immediately after injection two animals showed a rapid increase in locomotion, with frantic running and jumping resulting in many damaging collisions with the walls of the cage. These animals also showed what we describe as obstinate progression; on running across the cage and encountering a wall they tried to carry on in the same direction, making locomotory limb movements while pressing against the wall. In the first of these animals this frantic behaviour was interspersed with episodes of lying prostrate with twitching movements of the limbs, tongue rolling and opening and closing of the mouth. These two types of behaviour continued for about 1 h, after which the animal became prostrate and twitched continuously. After a further 4 h, twitching was suppressed with diazepam (3 mg/kg). The animal seemed normal after 24 h. The second animal showed essentially similar behaviour for about 40 min after which it became quiet and fell asleep. The remaining two animals showed vigorous, self-destructive movements, checking and unusual mouth and tongue movements for about 1 hr after injection, followed by a quiet somnolent phase (Ridley *et al.*, 1980a). These dramatic behavioural effects of apomorphine can be rapidly antagonised with 0.1-0.2 mg/kg haloperidol (Scraggs *et al.*, 1979).

When haloperidol was administered to otherwise untreated marmosets there was a dose-related decrease in locomotion, checking, general activities and contact with a corresponding increase in inactivity over the range 0-0.18 mg/kg. The animals sat quietly or slept at the higher dose.

2.6.2 *Assessment of cognitive function*

This section deals with the techniques used in this laboratory to assess the marmoset's ability to perform certain tasks involving cognitive skills. Although primates are employed in experiments using operant-conditioning paradigms where emphasis is laid on rates of responding or types of schedule able to maintain responding, we do not feel that primates offer advantages over rodents in this area. Almost all the significant advances in the investigation of primate cognitive ability (and effects of certain interventions thereon) have been achieved through the use of discrete trial discriminative training where animals try to solve problems trial by trial. Here it is accuracy of responding and not rate of responding which is of importance. Virtually all the early work and a large proportion of the contemporary work uses large Old World monkeys, but there is a growing interest in the use of smaller animals for experiments of this sort. Before discussing the variety of cognitive tasks employed in these investigations we will consider the apparatus and techniques of discrete trial discrimination training.

2.6.2.1 *Using operant apparatus.* Most types of rodent operant-conditioning apparatus (Skinner boxes) can be modified to accommodate a marmoset (see Fig. 2.6) and to present discrete trials. Banana-flavoured pellets (e.g. BRS/LVE, Beltsville, MD, USA) or freshly homogenised banana may be used as a food reward. The marmoset's temperamental disposition, however, makes this species less suitable than the rodent for certain types of schedule, and the separate positions of the stimulus lights, response levers and reward delivery system make discrete trial training in this apparatus more difficult for the animal than in the Wisconsin General Test Apparatus (see below). A naive animal, one that has never experienced an operant training system, will need to be 'shaped' before it can be tested in an experiment. The usual approach is to reward the animal for successive approximations to the correct response (lever pressing), making the criterion for reward more stringent on each approximation. For example, the animal will be put in the chamber and observed through the window. As it moves about the chamber it will be rewarded as it approaches the lever (this is done by manual override). Then, perhaps, it will be rewarded only when it touches the lever with a part of the body and, finally, only when it touches the lever with its hand. The lever will then be activated so that the animal is rewarded only when it presses the lever. Marmosets acquire the lever-pressing response after several daily training sessions, although care must be taken not to reward inappropriate responses otherwise the animal will learn bad, or 'superstitious' habits. Having acquired the response the animal can be trained to press in response to certain stimuli, e.g. to a light or a tone. In our labora-

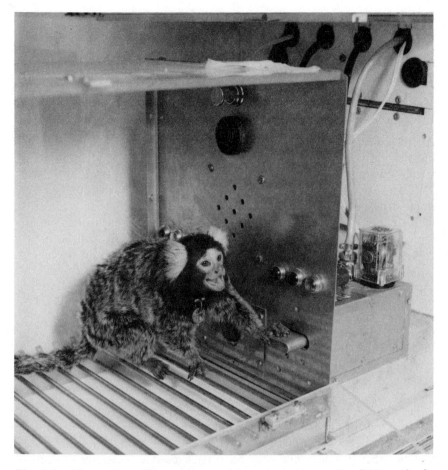

Fig. 2.6. Marmoset making a response in an operant apparatus (Skinner box). The chamber has been left open for photography.

tory we have tended to investigate trial-by-trial performance under certain drug conditions and have not been concerned with the more traditional aspects of operant training such as rate of lever pressing, which we will not discuss further. Complex schedules such as delayed spatial alternation may result in the development of superstitious behaviour; we have observed marmosets employ unusual methods of lever pressing. For example, one animal used its back legs, which may have represented an attempt to solve the problem in terms of body posture rather than choice of lever. Very occasionally animals may develop the habit of frantic jumping inside the chamber, probably in an attempt to escape. Under such circumstances it would be sensible to give the animal a prolonged rest and to alter the schedule. Food deprivation seems to make the situation worse; a food-deprived animal will often work faster but more frantically and less accurately, or will refuse to work at all. One of the advantages of using operant equipment for trial-by-trial perform-ance lies in the automatic way in which the stimuli are presented and the reward delivered, but in our experience the animals learn more quickly in the manually operated Wisconsin General Test Apparatus.

2.6.2.2 *Using Wisconsin General Test Apparatus (WGTA).* Possibly the most extensively used device for the neuropsychological study of primates is the Wisconsin General Test Apparatus designed by Harlow (1949). This is a structure in which the experimenter can present the monkey with single trials of a learning task and assess its trial-by-trial cumulative performance. It consists, essentially, of a large, cubical enclosure contain-ing a test board inset with small food wells. These wells can be baited with food and covered with various stimuli. The monkey in its cage is separated from the interior of the WGTA by an opaque shutter which the experimenter can open at the beginning of each trial. When the shutter is open, the animal can reach through the bars of its cage into the WGTA, and can displace a stimulus to claim the reward. After the trial is com-pleted, the shutter is closed and the experimenter can reload the wells through a trap door at the other end of the apparatus. The apparatus is arranged so that the animal cannot see the experimenter but the ex-perimenter can watch the animal during each trial through a one-way viewing system (see Figs. 2.7 and 2.8.).

The WGTA has been used mainly for large primates such as the rhesus monkey, but in our laboratory we have constructed several for use with marmosets. The performance of marmosets compares favourably with that of other primates and they have been used successfully in tests of learning, reversal learning, object preference and learning set formation (see below). We have used very small cubes of fresh banana as reward since this is a much preferred food for this species, though small cubes of apple or currants may be accepted. The banana-flavoured pellets men-tioned above may be suitable for some animals.

Shaping the marmoset for use in the WGTA is similar to shaping for the operant system. The animal is first presented with open, baited food wells and the stimuli are gradually moved over the wells on successive trials until they are completely covered. When the animal will respond to both stimuli (both are rewarded at this stage) and at both food wells, shaping is complete, and discrimination learning, where the reward is always put under one and the same stimulus, can begin. For stimuli we use small toy figures or 'junk' objects (pen-tops, paper clips, pencil sharpeners, bottle tops, etc.) about 5 cm in the largest dimension. Mar-

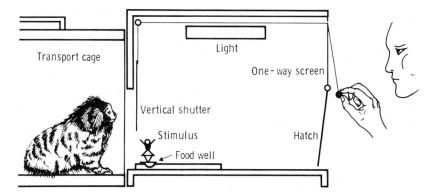

Fig. 2.7. Diagram of the Wisconsin General Test Apparatus (WGTA).

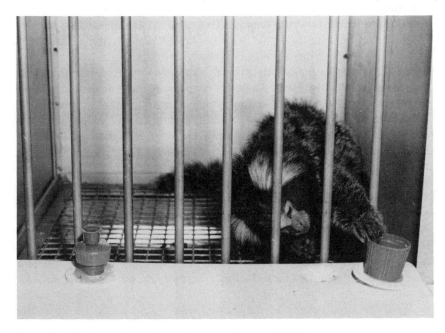

Fig. 2.8. A marmoset makes a response in the WGTA.

mosets can also be trained on simple pattern or colour discrimination (Miles, 1958). Although the retinal system of these animals has not been studied extensively, there is evidence that New World monkeys are equipped with a colour visual system which is anomalous with respect to other primates (Da Valois and Jacobs, 1968). Colour discrimination may be made partly on the basis of brightness rather than hue, and matching brightness for the human visual system may not be appropriate for the marmoset. Occasionally animals show strong idiosyncratic aversions to certain stimuli. Since this cannot be predicted in advance, experiments using junk objects should be designed to take this into account. In our experiments we assign junk objects at random and try to ensure that each animal meets each object only once during its experimental career. In order to ensure that the animal learns the discrimination on the basis of the stimulus association rather than because the reward is always on, say, the left, the left/right position of the stimuli is varied according to a 'pseudo-random' schedule. In one such schedule, described by Geller-mann (1933), the reward appears unpredictably on the left or right, though in each block of 10 trials it appears five times on each side. Unfortunately, marmosets, like the bigger primates, are not ashamed to cheat now and then. The experienced worker will have learnt not to give the animal any clues, other than the stimuli, on which to base its re-sponse. While the shutter is closed between trials, the animal may be listening to the sounds of the well being baited and the stimuli being moved about. Perhaps an over-committed worker might be tempted to groan slightly as he realises that the animal is about to displace the wrong stimulus and is then surprised when it changes its mind at the last minute. There are many ways of communicating information that will affect the monkey's behaviour, all of which must be identified and suppressed if the animal is going to perform adequately and respond only to the stimuli. Some workers use a 'white noise' generator to mask the sounds which are likely to interfere with the animal's behaviour; others find that a radio playing music will do just as well. A marmoset may also learn to wait for a short time where it last responded and then move to the other side. If the experimenter rebaits a repeated trial more quickly than he rearranges stimuli for an opposite trial, the animal will be able to predict where the next reward will be so care should be taken to maintain a relatively constant inter-trial interval. Marmosets are easily distracted by visual as well as auditory interference. The test cage should have opaque walls on all sides except facing the shutter. Sawdust should not be used on the floor of the cage otherwise the animal may spend a considerable time sifting through it.

We have found that it is not necessary to maintain strict food depriva-tion during these training sessions, and that a very hungry animal per-forms badly. A slight reduction in an animal's daily food provision can be of use in maintaining interest during the shaping procedure, but once an animal has been shaped, its natural enthusiasm for banana is usually adequate to ensure good performance. Our usual procedure is to feed the animal its normal daily diet after the day's training session is finished. On those occasions when an animal is performing poorly, bread or monkey chow might be substituted for banana in its diet for a day or two.

2.6.2.3 *The problem of criterion.* Training in a WGTA is usually continued until a predetermined criterion is reached. Commonly used criteria are 90 correct responses in 100 consecutive trials for tasks that require several days or weeks of training, or nine correct responses in ten consecutive trials for tasks that must be completed in one training session. We have used five consecutive correct responses as a very low criterion where more than one task has to be completed within one session, although this criterion has only limited suitability (see below). The choice of criterion is very important since it may profoundly affect the result of the experiment and subsequent experiments in the same animal. Choice of criterion depends on expected task difficulty (although to some extent task difficulty also depends on criterion, see below); the reason for conducting the training, e.g. intended retesting using the same or related tasks; and the sophistication of the animals. A naive animal should be trained to a criterion of 90/100 on its first task and to similar high criteria on the next few tasks in order to develop the habit of problem-solving. If this is not done, the animal is likely to develop a 'failure set', i.e. to approach all tasks as if they merely offer 50% reward. Similarly, an animal that fails to master a task in several hundred trials should be retrained to a fairly high criterion on an easy task before attempting another difficult task.

Roughly speaking, 'overtraining' may be said to have occurred where the number of trials in criterion greatly exceeds the number of trials up to criterion (the learning score). Thus in a group of animals learning the same task to the same criterion, some animals may be 'overtrained' and others not. Constantly adjusted criteria based on projected learning scores can be devised (Ettlinger and Rashbass, 1976) but do not totally overcome problems arising from individual differences in learning ability. A degree of overtraining is likely to improve retention and learning of similar tasks; an easy task learnt to 90/100 may be retained indefinitely. However, the improvement in reversal learning following overtraining which is seen in rodents (the overtraining reversal effect), has not been observed in primates (Sutherland and Mackintosh, 1971).

Figure 2.9 shows the learning scores for successive 90% criteria for a group of twelve marmosets learning a simple visual discrimination to 90 correct responses in 100 trials. It can be seen that after the criterion of 9/10 which is reached in less than 40 trials, criteria of 18/20 up to 45/50 are equally difficult, 54/60 and 63/70 are slightly harder but 72/80 up to 90/100 are reached slightly earlier. Where an animal performs at ~90% correct, successive 90% criteria are reached simultaneously, since for every ten trials, one error is made on average. Where the learning score decreases for successive 90% criteria, the animal is performing at about 100% correct. In most cases learning scores do not increase if 90% criteria above 18/20 are used. This is not the case for 'consecutive' criteria.

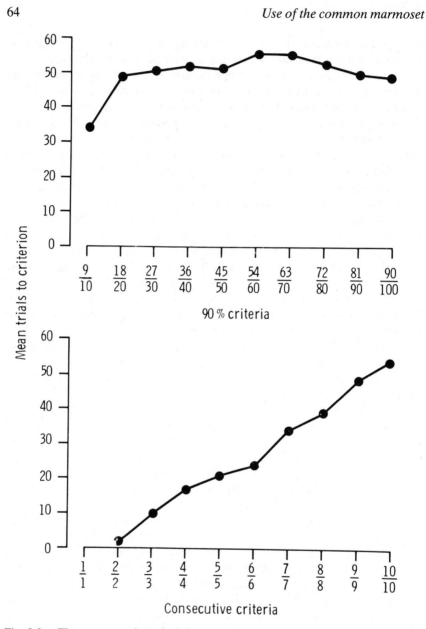

Fig. 2.9.   The mean number of trials to reach successive 90% criteria (upper) and successive 'consecutive correct' criteria (lower) in a visual discrimination task ($N = 12$ and 10 animals respectively).

Figure 2.9 also shows that scores at which successive 'consecutive' criteria (i.e. 2/2, 3/3, etc.) are reached increase approximately linearly. Thus 7/7 is roughly equivalent to 9/10, and 9/9 to between 18/20 and 81/90. Consecutive criteria of 10/10 and higher may be expected to be harder than any 90% criterion if, as is suggested by the data, animals tend to perform at never much better than 90% correct.

Although in a binomial experiment five correct responses in a *total* of five trials (with the probability of a correct response $= 0.5$) has a probability of $P = 0.03$, and nine correct responses in a *total* of ten trials has a probability of $P = 0.01$, a more important assumption of 'learning' in the animal is the expected number of trials that would be performed before such a criterion sequence might occur *by chance*. In order to test this we have performed a computer simulation over 200 runs each for several criteria. On average 55 trials occurred before five consecutive correct responses were made by chance and 225 trials before seven consecutive corrects or 9/10 correct responses were achieved by chance. The number of trials before higher 90% criteria were reached were inestimably high by our system. A criterion of five consecutive correct responses is only appropriate where several, very easy tasks with expected learning scores well below 50 have to be performed by an animal in one day.

Groups of animals may be compared using a low criterion so long as the learning scores of the 'unimpaired' group are very low. Learning scores of 50 or more in the other group may be taken as evidence of impairment but not necessarily of learning. These arguments only apply if animals begin a task by performing at chance level. In reversal, for example, a different relation of criterion to learning score may be tolerable.

2.6.2.4 *Applications of discrete trial training methods.* Discrete trial discrimination training can be used to assess almost any cognitive process from the detection of sensory thresholds to the development of concepts in primates (Meyer, 1971; Ridley and Ettlinger, 1976). It can be used in any sensory modality although visual testing predominates. Auditory discrimination (Weiskrantz and Mishkin, 1958) and tactile testing including somatosensory and proprioceptive (weight and joint-position) testing are feasible with some modifications to the WGTA (see, for example, Ridley and Ettlinger, 1978). Even olfactory testing has been achieved, although without great elegance (Brown, 1963). A comprehensive demonstration of how the judicious choice of tasks can be used to specify the precise nature of an observed impairment is given by work on inferotemporal lesions in monkeys (see Gross, 1972, for review).

Although not used extensively, marmosets compare well with other primates on many tests, and we see no reason why most tasks should not be attempted in this species. Tasks involving a delay between stimulus presentation and response are particularly difficult but by no means impossible for marmosets (Miles, 1957; Weight *et al.*, 1980). We have found delayed alternation to be difficult (Baker *et al.*, 1982). Tasks involving delay are typically affected by frontal lesions (Warren and Akert, 1964). The relative difficulty exhibited by marmosets on these tasks may reflect their lowly position in the primate phylogenetic tree since the expansion of the frontal granular cortex is the most recent evolutionary development in the brain.

The ability of monkeys to perceive and attend to visual dimensions can be tested by the systematic choice of stimuli consisting of different colours, shapes, patterns, sizes, etc., in varying combinations. Ability to form and remember reward associations can be tested by *concurrent* learning where several pairs of stimuli are presented on successive trials until all the tasks have been learnt (Cowey and Gross, 1970), or by serial reversal learning (Manning, 1972). The inability to dissolve a reward association is demonstrated by perseverative (worse than chance) performance on the early trials of reversal learning (Ridley *et al.*, 1981c). More recently it has been shown that a more sensitive measure of the ability to recognise and form reward associations is given by trial unique object discrimination tasks (Gaffan, 1974; Spiegler and Mishkin, 1981). On these tasks recognition is demonstrated by the ability of the monkey to choose the novel object when presented with a choice between a novel object and a 'familiar' object encountered on the previous trial. Reward association is demonstrated by the ability of the monkey to choose the novel object if the familiar object was *unrewarded* on the previous trial but the familiar object if it was *rewarded* on the previous trial. Other short-term cognitive skills requiring retention of information for 5–30 s, but using repeated presentation of the same stimuli, can be demonstrated by tests of delayed response, delayed alternation and delayed matching-to-sample (Warren and Akert, 1964).

Long-term retention has usually been measured in the past by the use of saving scores:

$$\text{saving score} = \frac{\text{original learning score-retention score}}{\text{original learning score}} \times 100\%$$

This measure, however, has certain disadvantages. Learning scores and retention scores are not strictly comparable since on retention testing the stimuli may not be novel, i.e. unrecognised, even if the reward association is not retained. Novelty may in itself affect performance. Gross distortion may in itself affect performance, and may occur if the learning scores are very low since one unfortunate error can double the learning or retention score. Mahut *et al.* (1981) have found that the difference between reversal scores and retention scores on successive days of the same task gives a sound measure of the amount of reward association carried over from the previous day. We have found comparison of 24-h reversal and retention scores of different tasks to be a good measure of memory for reward association in the marmoset, suitable for assessing the effects of drugs on encoding and retrieval aspects of long-term memory. The formation of learning sets is a most important concept in primate learning (Harlow, 1949). A learning set can be said to have been formed when an animal performs reliably better than chance on the second and subsequent trials of any discrimination task of one type even though the stimulus objects have not been encountered before. Marmosets form learning sets for object discrimination (Miles and Meyer, 1956) and reversal learning (Cotterman *et al.*, 1956) but with considerably less facility than macaques. In our experience, after the first two or three discrimination tasks during which learning scores fall dramatically, the marmoset's learning ability does not improve for at least the next 100 tasks. In one recent series of experiments (Ridley *et al.*, 1981d) involving about 100 separate object discriminations, the mean learning score on the first experiment was not different from that on the last experiment for the saline control conditions. This stable level of performance over time makes it possible to study, for example, the effects of different doses of drugs in the same animal without undue interference from overtraining, although in practice we always present doses in ascending and then descending order and sum the results at each dose.

Whereas in rodents training on one task may interfere with training on another (e.g. if a shift from position to visual discrimination is involved), in monkeys training on any task except alternation is likely to facilitate further training on almost any other task. This is because almost all tasks involve a strategy of 'win–stay', 'lose–shift' except alternation which requires a 'win–shift', 'lose–stay' strategy. Thus protracted training contributes not only to specific learning set formation, e.g. reversal or object learning set, but also to a global 'win–stay' set (Warren, 1966; Sutherland and Mackintosh, 1971). This multidimensional set formation separates the primate from the rodent in cognitive mechanism. Despite the fact that we have found that marmosets form complete learning sets only slowly, we have found a uniform lack of interference between tasks. Some interference is found in the early stages of serial reversal learning but this is largely overcome after about 5–10 reversals, after which relearning and reversal learning scores are similar (Ridley *et al.*, 1981c). When learning two consecutive object discriminations, there is no tendency for the second task to be either easier or more difficult than the first for undrugged animals (Ridley *et al.*, 1981d). Similarly, we have found not only no difference in task difficulty between colour discrimination and grey-shape discrimination, but also no difference between colour following shape and colour-first discrimination or shape following colour and shape-first discrimination in undrugged animals (Baker *et al.*, 1982). In a further experiment we found no difference in overall difficulty between position discrimination and object discrimination learning using the same stimuli, but a significant difficulty ($P < 0.005$) on changing from one rule to another compared with retention from the day before. Thus some interference is found on this non-reversal task, and on reversal learning where the same stimuli are used in both tasks, but not between tasks using different stimuli.

It can be seen that, despite its small size and lowly position in the primate hierarchy, the marmoset is capable of very sophisticated cognitive processes. It is our opinion that the major constraint on the use of discrete trial testing lies more with the ingenuity and patience of the experimenter than with the potential of either monkey or apparatus.

2.6.2.5 Studies on the role of catecholamines in cognitive functions. We have used the methods described above to study the effects of catecholamine-acting drugs on cognitive function in the marmoset.

Using the rodent operant apparatus we have shown that, over a dose range of 0.2–1.2 mg/kg, amphetamine disrupted the marmoset's ability to perform a successive go–no go visual discrimination but did not affect performance of a simultaneous version of the same task (Ridley *et al.*, 1980b). Nor did the drug affect a successive go here – go there discrimination where a response was required on each type of trial (Ridley *et al.*, 1980d). After amphetamine, marmosets were also mildly impaired on a delayed response version of the same task (Weight *et al.*, 1980). From these results it was concluded that amphetamine affects the *performance* of tasks requiring a degree of response inhibition.

Using the WGTA we found that animals treated with amphetamine were not impaired at performing a well-learnt discrimination task, nor at relearning a task which they had performed last on the previous day. They were, however, severely impaired at learning the reversal of a task which they had just performed to a predetermined criterion (Ridley *et al.*, 1981c). This effect was not seen if the animals were pretreated with the dopamine-blocking drug, haloperidol. In two further experiments it was found that marmosets treated with amphetamine were unable to relinquish either an idiosyncratic or experimentally induced object preference (Ridley *et al.*, 1981a,b). From this it was concluded that amphetamine disrupts the *learning* of tasks where the inhibition of a previously acquired reward association is necessary.

We have also investigated the role of noradrenaline in cognitive performance using the α-noradrenergic blocking drug, aceperone (Janssen *et al.*, 1967). Animals injected with aceperone were found to be severely and consistently impaired at learning the first task of each test session, and to be impaired on new, and repeated, reversal learning. They were not, however, impaired at learning another similar task in each test session or at performing a well-learnt task. We have interpreted these rather complicated results as evidence for a dysfunction in the processes required for association formation which can be compensated for by suitable priming or practice (Ridley *et al.*, 1981d).

This section is not intended to be a comprehensive account of the experiments on catecholamine involvement in cognitive processes carried out in this laboratory. For such an account the reader is referred to the original papers. It is hoped, however, that it will illustrate the way in which the techniques described in this chapter can be used to elucidate such an involvement. These lines of enquiry are being extended to investigate the effects of centrally acting drugs injected into discrete brain areas and are part of the work of this laboratory on schizophrenia and dementia.

References

Annett, L.E., Ridley, R.M., Gamble, S.J. and Baker, H.F. (1983). Behavioural effects of intracerebral amphetamine in the marmoset. *Psychopharmacol.* **81**, 18–23

Baker, H.F. and Ridley, R.M. (1979). Increased HVA levels in primate ventricular CSF following amphetamine administration. *Brain Res.* **167**, 206–9.

Baker, H.F., Ridley, R.M., Haystead, T.A.J. and Crow, T.J. (1982). Further consideration of the learning impairment after aceperone in the marmoset: effects of the drug on shape and colour discrimination and on an alternation task. *Pharmacol. Biochem. Behav.* **18**, 701–4.

Brown, T.S. (1963). Olfactory and visual discrimination in monkeys after selective lesions of the temporal lobe. *J. comp. physiol. Psychol.* **56**, 764–8.

Cotterman, T.E., Meyer, D.R. and Wickens, D.D. (1956). Discrimination reversal learning in marmosets. *J. comp. physiol. Psychol.* **49**, 539–41.

Cowey, A. and Gross, C.G. (1970). Effects of foveal prestriate and inferotemporal lesions on visual discrimination by rhesus monkeys. *Exp. Brain Res.* **11**, 128–44.

De Valois, R.L. and Jacobs, G.H. (1968). Primate colour vision. The macaque and squirrel monkey differ in their colour vision and in the physiology of their visual system. *Science* **162**, 533–40.

Ellison, G., Nielson, E.B. and Lyon, M. (1981). Animal model of psychosis; hallucinatory behaviour in monkeys during the late stage of continuous amphetamine intoxication. *J. Psychiat. Res.* **16**, 13–22.

Ettlinger, G. and Rashbass, C. (1976). Adjusting the amount of overtraining to the difficulty of discrimination learning. *Neuropsychologia* **14**, 257–60.

Flecknell, P.A., Parry, R.P., Ridley, R.M., Baker, H.F., Bowes, P. and Needham, J.R. (1982). Respiratory disease associated with parainfluenza-I

(Sendai) virus in a colony of marmosets (*Callithrix jacchus*). *Lab. Anim.* **17**, 111–13

Gaffan, D. (1974). Recognition impaired and association intact in the memory of monkeys after transection of the fornix. *J. comp. physiol. Psychol.* **86**, 1100–9.

Gellermann, L.W. (1933). Chance orders of alternating stimuli in visual discrimination experiments. *J. Genet. Psychol.* **42**, 206–8.

Gross, C.G. (1972). Inferotemporal cortex and vision. In *Progress in Physiological Psychology*, Vol. 5 (E. Stellar and J.M. Sprague, Eds), 77–123, Academic Press, New York.

Harlow, H.F. (1949). The formation of learning sets. *Psychol. Rev.* **56**, 51–65.

Harlow, H.F. (1962). Development of the second and third affectional systems in macaque monkeys. In *Research Approaches to Psychiatric Problems* (T.T. Tourlentes, Ed.), Grune and Stratton, New York.

Hearn, J.P. and Burden, F.J. (1979). 'Collaborative' rearing of marmoset triplets. *Lab. Anim.* **13**, 131–3.

Hodgen, G.D., Wolfe, L.G., Ogden, J.D., Adams, M.R., Descalzi, C.C. and Hildebrand, D.F. (1976). Diagnosis of pregnancy in marmosets: haemagglutination—inhibition test and radioimmunoassay for urinary chorionic gonadotrophin. *Lab. Anim. Sci.* **26**, 224–9.

Howie, J.M. (1978). Code of Practice for the Prevention of Infection in Clinical Laboratories. Report of a Working Party Chaired by J.M. Howie. HMSO, London.

Hunt, R.D., Anderson, M.P. and Chalifoux, L.V. (1978). Spontaneous infectious diseases of marmosets. *Primate Med.* **10**, 239–53.

Ingram, J.C. (1975). Husbandry and observation methods of a breeding colony of marmosets (*Callithrix jacchus*) for behavioural research. *Lab. Anim.* **9**, 249–59.

Janssen, P., Niemegeers, C., Schellekens, K. and Lenaerts, F. (1967). Is it possible to predict the clinical effects of neuroleptic drugs (major tranquillisers) from animal data? IV. An improved experimental design for measuring the inhibitory effects of neuroleptic drugs on amphetamine-or apomorphine-induced chewing and agitation in rats. *Arzneimittel-Forsch.* **17**, 841–54.

Joseph, M.H., Baker, H.F. and Ridley, R.M. (1981). Analyses of CSF amine metabolites and precursors including tryptophan, 5HIAA and HVA by HPLC using EC detection: the effect of probenecid studied in primates. In *Central Transmitter Turnover* (C.J. Pycock and P.V. Taberner, Eds), 162–7, Croom Helm, London.

Köhler, W. (1925). *The Mentality of Apes*, Pelican, Harmondsworth (published 1957)

Levy, B.M. and Mircovic, R.R. (1971). An epizootic of measles in a marmoset colony. *Lab. Anim. Care* **21**, 33–9.

Lunn, S.F., Hobson, B.M. and Hearn, J.P. (1979). Pregnancy diagnosis in the common marmoset (*Callithrix jacchus jacchus*). *Folia primatol.* **32**, 200–6.

Mahut, H., Moss, M. and Zola-Morgan, S. (1981). Retention deficits after combined amygdalo-hippocampal and selective hippocampal resections in the monkey. *Neuropsychologia* **19**, 201–25.

Manning, F.J. (1972). Serial reversal learning by monkeys with inferotemporal or foveal prestriate lesions. *Physiology Behav.* **8**, 177–81.

Meyer, D.R. (1971). The habits and concepts of monkeys. In *Cognitive Processes in Non-human Primates* (L.E. Jarrard, Ed.), 83–102, Academic Press, New York.

Miles, R.C. (1957). Delayed-response learning in the marmoset and the macaque.

J. comp. physiol. Psychol. **50**, 352–5.

Miles, R.C. (1958). Colour vision in the marmoset. *J. comp. physiol. Psychol.* **51**, 152–4.

Miles, R.C. and Meyer, D.R. (1956). Learning sets in marmosets. *J. comp. physiol. Psychol.* **49**, 219–22.

Mishkin, M. (1978). Memory in monkeys severely impaired by combined but not by separate removal of amygdala and hippocampus. *Nature* **273**, 297–8.

Mishkin, M., Spiegler, B.J., Saunders, R.C. and Malamut, B.L. (1982). An animal model of global amnesia. In *Alzheimer's Disease: a Review of Progress* (S. Corkin, K.L. Davis, J.H. Growden, E. Usdin and R.J. Wurtman, Eds), 235–47, Raven Press, New York.

Perkins, F.T. and O'Donoghue, P.N. (1969). Hazards of handling simians. *Proceedings of the 29th Symposium, Permanent Section of Microbiological Standardisation of the International Association of Microbiological Societies*, Laboratory Animals Ltd, London.

Phillips, I.R. and Grist, S.M. (1975). The use of transabdominal palpation to determine the course of pregnancy in the marmoset (*Callithrix jacchus*). *J. Reprod. Fert.* **43**, 103–8.

Poole, T.B. and Evans, R.G. (1982). Reproduction, infant survival and productivity of a colony of common marmosets (*Callithrix jacchus jacchus*). *Lab. Anim.* **16**, 88–97.

Randrup, A. and Munkvad, I. (1967). Stereotyped activities produced by amphetamine in several animal species and man. *Psychopharmacologia* **11**, 300–10.

Ridley R.M. and Baker H.F. (1982). Stereotypy in monkeys and humans. *Psychol. Med.* **12**, 61–72

Ridley R.M. and Baker H.F. (1983). Is there a relationship between social isolation, cognitive inflexibility and behavioural stereotypy? An analysis of the effects of amphetamine in the marmoset. In *Ethopharmacology: Primate Models of Neuropsychiatric Disorders* (K.A. Miczek, Ed.), 101–35 Alan R. Liss, New York.

Ridley, R.M. and Ettlinger, G. (1976). Impaired tactile learning retention after removals of the second somatic sensory projection cortex SII in the monkey. *Brain Res.* **109**, 656–60.

Ridley, R.M. and Ettlinger, G. (1978). Further evidence of impaired tactile learning after removals of the second somatic sensory cortex (SII) in the monkey. *Exp. Brain Res.* **31**, 475–88.

Ridley, R.M., Baker, H.F. and Scraggs, P.R. (1979a). The time course of the behavioural effects of amphetamine and their reversal by haloperidol in a primate species. *Biol. Psychiat.* **14**, 753–65.

Ridley, R.M., Scraggs, P.R. and Baker, H.F. (1979b). Modification of the behavioural effects of amphetamine by a GABA agonist in a primate species. *Psychopharmacology* **64**, 197–200.

Ridley, R.M., Baker, H.F. and Crow, T.J. (1980a). Behavioural effects of amphetamines and related stimulants: the importance of species differences as demonstrated by a study in the marmoset. In *Amphetamines and Related Stimulants: Chemical, Biological, Clinical and Sociological Aspects* (J. Caldwell, Ed.), 97–116, CRC Press, Florida.

Ridley, R.M., Baker, H.F. and Weight, M.L. (1980b). Amphetamine disrupts successive but not simultaneous visual discrimination in the monkey. *Psychopharmacology* **67**, 241–4.

Ridley, R.M., Scraggs, P.R. and Baker, H.F. (1980c). The effects of metoclopramide, sulpiride and the stereoisomers of baclofen on amphetamine-induced behaviour in the marmoset. *Biol. Psychiat.* **15**, 265–74.

Ridley, R.M., Weight, M.L., Haystead, T.A.J. and Baker, H.F. (1980d). 'Go here — Go there' performance after amphetamine: the importance of the response requirement in successive discrimination. *Psychopharmacology* **69**, 271–3.

Ridley, R.M., Baker, H.F. and Haystead, T.A.J. (1981a). Perseverative behaviour after amphetamine: dissociation of response tendency from reward association. *Psychopharmacol.* **75**, 283–6.

Ridley, R.M., Haystead, T.A.J. and Baker, H.F. (1981b). An involvement of dopamine in higher order choice mechanisms in the monkey. *Psychopharmacol.* **72**, 173–7.

Ridley, R.M., Haystead, T.A.J. and Baker, H.F. (1981c). An analysis of visual object reversal learning in the marmoset after amphetamine and haloperidol. *Pharmacol. Biochem. Behav.* **14**, 345–51.

Ridley, R.M., Haystead, T.A.J., Baker, H.F. and Crow, T.J. (1981d). A new approach to the role of noradrenaline in learning: problem-solving in the marmoset after α-noradrenergic receptor blockade. *Pharmacol. Biochem. Behav.* **14**, 849–55.

Scraggs, P.R. and Ridley, R.M. (1978). Behavioural effects of amphetamine in a small primate: relative potencies of the *d*- and *l*-isomers. *Psychopharmacology* **59**, 243–5.

Scraggs, P.R. and Ridley, R.M. (1979). The effect of dopamine and noradrenaline blockade on amphetamine-induced behaviour in the marmoset. *Psychopharmacology* **62**, 41–5.

Scraggs, P.R., Baker, H.F. and Ridley, R.M. (1979). Interaction of apomorphine and haloperidol: effects on locomotion and other behaviour in the marmoset. *Psychopharmacology* **66**, 41–3.

Shimwell, M., Warrington, B.F. and Fowler, J.S.L. (1979). Dietary habits relating to 'wasting marmoset syndrome' (WMS). *Lab. Anim.* **13**, 139–42.

Spiegler, B.J. and Mishkin, M. (1981). Evidence for the sequential participation of inferior temporal cortex and amygdala in the acquisition of stimulus–reward associations. *Behav. Brain Res.* **3**, 303–17.

Stein, F.J., Lewis, D.H., Stott, G.G. and Sis, R.F. (1981). Acute gastric dilatation in common marmosets. *Lab. Anim. Sci.* **31**, 522–3.

Stephan, H., Baron, G. and Schwerdtfeger, W.K. (1980). *The Brain of the Common Marmoset (Callithrix jacchus): a Stereotaxic Atlas*, Springer-Verlag, Berlin.

Stevenson, M.F. (1976). Maintenance and breeding of the common marmoset (*C. jacchus*) with notes on hand-rearing. *Int. Zoo Yearbook* **16**, 110–16.

Stevenson, M.F. and Poole, T.B. (1976). An ethogram of the common marmoset (*C. jacchus*): general behavioural repertoire. *Anim. Behav.* **24**, 428–51.

Sutherland, N.S. and Mackintosh, N.J. (1971). *Mechanisms of Animal Discrimination Learning*, 432–3, Academic Press, London.

Warren, J.M. (1966). Reversal learning and the formation of learning sets by cats and rhesus monkeys. *J. comp. physiol. Psychol.* **61**, 421–8.

Warren, J.M. and Akert, K. (1964). *The Frontal Granular Cortex and Behaviour*, McGraw-Hill, New York.

Weight, M.L., Ridley, R.M. and Baker, H.F. (1980). The effect of amphetamine on delayed response performance in the monkey. *Pharmacol., Biochem. Behav.* **12**, 861–4.

Weiskrantz, L. and Mishkin, M. (1958). Effects of temporal and frontal cortical lesions on auditory discrimination in monkeys. *Brain* **81**, 406–14.

Ziegler, T.E., Stein, F.J., Sis, R.F., Coleman, M.S. and Green, J.H. (1981). Supplemental feeding of marmoset *Callithrix jacchus* triplets. *Lab. Anim. Sci.* **31**, 194–5.

3 *David G. Cunningham Owens*

Practical problems in evaluating involuntary motor activity in schizophrenic patients

3.1 Introduction

The problems of clinical psychiatric research are inextricably rooted in the nature of the conditions with which the specialty deals. With the exception of organic brain disease, objective measures for validating the features that form diagnostic categories are not available and no psycho-pathological feature can be shown to be pathognomonic of any specific condition. Diagnosis, for instance that of schizophrenia, is based on the exercise of judgement as to the significance of a particular constellation of features to a particular personal and historical setting.

This was very much the position in general medicine a century ago. The understanding of bodily function in health and disease that we now have was made possible by the development of objective techniques of investigation. The continuing lack of such techniques applicable to psychiatry has held the specialty at the largely descriptive level at which it still operates.

One might therefore suppose that a clear-cut neurological syndrome, characterised by gross signs of motor dysfunction, would be the answer to a research psychiatrist's prayers. This alas has not quite proved to be the case. The literature on involuntary movement disorder occurring in patients exposed to neuroleptic (antipsychotic) medication is confusing. Evaluating the same evidence, some authorities have been 'thoroughly convinced' of the link between these drugs and involuntary movements (Marsden *et al.*, 1975), and others remain sceptical (Turek, 1975; Crow *et al.*, 1981).

Some of this confusion has arisen for reasons that are clear. Studies of the 'look and see' variety dominated the early work in this field. By 'looking' at heterogeneous patient samples using unstandardised procedures, they 'saw' different things. It is only in the last decade that the importance of a more systematic approach to methodology has been widely recognised in the study of involuntary movements.

The introduction of standardised examination and recording techniques and the use of operational criteria in defining homogeneous populations only tackle the obvious sources of variation. Unfortunately, the characteristics of the clinical features being studied make discrepant findings all too likely. Involuntary movements in man are the subject of many subtle influences, the assessment of which is most difficult in just those patients who form the focus of research interest.

It is not the purpose of this chapter to provide a literature review or an evaluation of assessment methods (see Gardos *et al.*, 1977; APA Task Force Report, 1979: summarised 1980; Jeste and Wyatt, 1981; Kane and Smith, 1982). Its purpose is simple, if presumptuous: to illustrate, by way of one clinical example, the sorts of problem encountered in studying patient samples. The example of involuntary movement disorder has been chosen because it is an area previously discussed in relation to animal work. It is in addition an area which well illustrates how a problem, apparently simple in abstraction, can become infinitely more complex when transposed to patients.

The following is based on the author's experience of examining several hundred chronic schizophrenics for involuntary movements (Owens *et al.*, 1982) using two standardised recording instruments, the Abnormal Involuntary Movement Scale or AIMS (Guy, 1976; see appendix 3.1) and the Simpson Dyskinesia Rating Scale (Simpson *et al.*, 1979; see appendix 3.2). Before proceeding, however, it is necessary to consider briefly the concept and clinical features to be discussed.

3.1.1 *The concept of tardive dyskinesia*

Spontaneous involuntary movements have long been known to neurologists, forming as they do an integral part of the symptomatology of a number of organic central nervous system disorders. For the most part, these disorders are uncommon, poorly understood, largely untreatable and usually progressive. Although detailed descriptions of the patterns of movement disorders found in these conditions have been available since the last century, systematic study of spontaneous movements is a recent development, largely prompted by the reported association between abnormal movements and administration of neuroleptic drugs.

Soon after their introduction, it was recognised that neuroleptics could produce neurological disturbance. A bradykinetic, Parkinson-like syndrome characterised by poverty of movement was described, usually emerging days to weeks after commencement of treatment (Hall *et al.*, 1956). Acute, often dramatic, neurological episodes were also reported, involving particularly head and neck posture and facial expression (Ayd, 1961; Melvin, 1962). These were not considered serious as they were apparently readily reversible and rarely interfered with management. In the 1960s, however, it was suggested that longer-term treatment with these preparations led to the development of a syndrome of involuntary movements that might not be reversible (Uhrbrand and Faurbye, 1960). The concept was formulated of 'neuroleptic-caused movement disorder', or 'tardive dyskinesia', the word 'tardive' being used to emphasise that the onset occurred later in the course of treatment than the other known neurological sequelae (Faurbye *et al.*, 1964).

This concept has become widened over the years in all its essentials. Although neuroleptics were the original — and remain *the* major — source of concern, many other types of preparation have been implicated (APA Task Force Report, 1979): the duration of treatment necessary for movements to be considered tardive has varied from 2 years down to 3 months: and the movements qualifying for 'dyskinesia' in this context have ranged from orofacial only to any movement in any body part. This generalisation and lack of clarity regarding the essentials of the concept undoubtedly account for some of the confusion referred to previously.

The idea of 'neuroleptic-caused movement disorder' is of more than theoretical interest. The efficacy of these drugs in the management of psychoses, especially schizophrenia, is established (Davis, 1975) and they are widely prescribed internationally. 'Tardive dyskinesia' is possibly the most frequently diagnosed iatrogenic disorder of the nervous system (Paulson, 1981). As an iatrogenic disorder, there are serious medico-legal implications, particularly in the United States.

3.1.2 *The clinical features*
The characteristic clinical picture is the buccomasticatory lingual (BML) triad (Marsden *et al.*, 1975; APA Task Force Report, 1979). Coarse vermicular movements of the tongue without its displacement are thought to be the earliest manifestations but are easily missed. Choreoathetoid lingual movements inside the dental margin are followed by sweeping movements of the tongue in and around the bucco-gingival space, giving the appearance of sucking a sweet ('bon-bon' sign). Eventually jerky, irregular — and later more sustained — extrusions of the tongue from the mouth, usually at the angles, follow ('fly-catcher' sign). These movements are associated with varying degrees of chewing, grinding jaw movements, and pursing, puckering and smacking activity of the lips and perioral musculature.

The BML triad can be accompanied by involuntary periorbital activity and movements in both upper and lower extremities. These are usually the rapid, jerky uncoordinated movements referred to as chorea and/or the slower, more sinuous movements of athetosis. Involvement of the large antigravity muscles of posture (often referred to descriptively as copulatory movements) can give the appearance of activity in the whole body.

Although the above implies a step-wise evolution of the clinical features, this is still by no means clear. One of the major diagnostic dilemmas relates to the great variability of symptom patterns, one determinant of which is likely to be the patient's age. Younger patients, especially children and adolescents, may for example be more prone to peripheral movements (Marsden *et al.*, 1975; APA Task Force Report, 1979). However, the exact relationship between the individual components of the syndrome and their evolution remains to be established.

3.2 **Problems inherent in the type of condition**

3.2.1 *The definition of dyskinesia*
The word 'dyskinesia' has a long history but was not widely used prior to its introduction in the context of drug aetiology. Strictly speaking, it is the generic neurological term for 'any abnormal kinesis'. Hence, choreoathetoid movements, jerks and twitches of tic-like or myoclonic type and even

tremors are, by this usage, dyskinesias. In the context of putative drug aetiology, however, clinical descriptions frequently emphasise or consider exclusively, the BML component of abnormality, implying a restricted understanding of 'dyskinesia' in this setting. Some authors have proposed definitions which are quite specific (Crane and Naranjo, 1971) and thereby underline this limited usage, when drugs are accepted as the cause of involuntary movements.

Differences in conceptualisation of this type can be seen behind the two rating scales referred to previously. The AIMS, for example, specifically excludes tremor, which some authorities have stated is not a feature of the 'tardive dyskinesia' syndrome (Marsden *et al.*, 1975). It is furthermore strongly biased towards facial abnormality, devoting four of its seven items to this area (appendix 3.1). The Simpson Scale on the other hand reserves specific items for rating tremor, and only 16 of its 43 items concentrate on facial movements (appendix 3.2).

Therefore, at the outset it must be decided whether a broad or a narrow concept of 'dyskinesia' is to be applied. The answer to this question should determine the recording technique to be used — rather than vice versa. The prevalence of abnormality found will in large part depend on the breadth of the concept adopted, and differences of this type certainly contribute to the wide discrepancies in prevalence reported in the literature. In our own work, taking a 'moderate' severity criterion (i.e. considering those with at least moderate abnormality), the Simpson Scale produced a prevalence of movement disorder that was 17% higher than the AIMS (Fig. 3.1; see also Owens *et al.*, 1982).

3.2.2 *Dyskinesia, mannerism or stereotypy?*

Repetitious, co-ordinated and apparently purposeless movements are commonly seen in chronic psychiatric patients, especially the mentally subnormal and those with chronic schizophrenia. Great stress was laid on these by the early descriptive psychiatrists, particularly Eugen Bleuler. Following this clinical tradition, movements which represent 'striking alterations of ordinary activities' (Bleuler, 1950) and to which subconscious 'meaning' may possibly be attributed, are referred to as mannerisms. When they are more rudimentary and apparently non-goal directed (and defy the best psychodynamic endeavours), they are called stereotypies. However, no clear, acceptable definition or classification of this .type of abnormality exists, and it represents a neglected area of research interest. Whether 'mannerisms' and 'stereotypies' can or should be separated is unclear, and where such movements stand in relation to 'dyskinesias' is unknown.

Most work on such motor abnormalities adopts an ethological approach to aetiology (Kramer and McKinney, 1979) and cites animal work, espe-

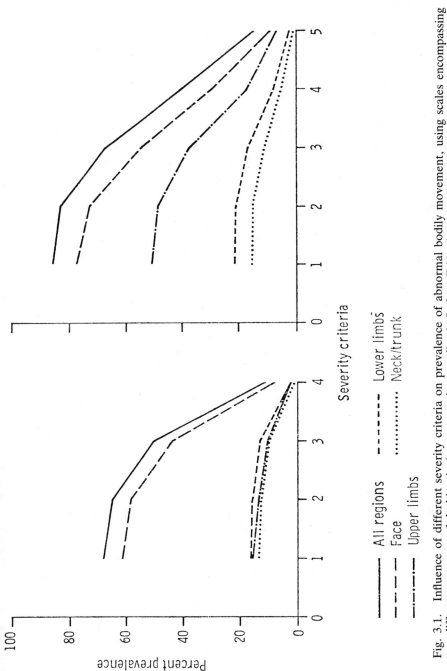

Fig. 3.1. Influence of different severity criteria on prevalence of abnormal bodily movement, using scales encompassing two different concepts of dyskinesia (see text and appendices). Left: AIMS, right: Rockland (Simpson *et al.*, 1979).

cially with primates, to confirm the belief that they represent a general behavioural reaction to confinement (or in animals, to captivity) (Randrup and Munkvad, 1967). Their function is suggested as being the vague but widely quoted one of 'tension reduction' (Boice and Kraemer, 1981). This may be reasonable if agreement could be reached as to when a particular movement is 'stereotypic' as opposed to 'dyskinetic'. A behavioural psychologist might consider crossing/uncrossing of the legs when sitting to be 'stereotyped' abnormality, yet this is item 38 in the 'Tardive (i.e. neuroleptic-caused) Dyskinesia' Rating Scale of Simpson *et al*. On the other hand, such activity may be disregarded in a general neurological clinic. Psychologists have described as a common stereotypy something referred to as '"in-place" walking', occurring with the patient both standing and seated (Boice and Kraemer, 1981). This sounds suspiciously like what psychiatrists and neurologists would diagnose as tasikinesia and akathisia respectively (Crane and Naranjo, 1971), features they would have no hesitation in attributing to neuroleptic drugs.

It remains to be seen whether mannerisms/stereotypies are truly involuntary in the sense that chorea and athetosis are understood as involuntary — that is, determined by some permanent biochemical or structural brain change, possibly in the striatum — or whether they are nothing more than acquired bad habits — the stylised idiosyncrasies of movement accentuated by an impoverished environment.

As is so often the case the answer will probably incorporate elements of both these views. The practical importance of the distinction is that, at the level of our present knowledge, motor activity believed to be manneristic/stereotypic should not be recorded on scales devised to score 'tardive dyskinesia'. Movements like these are known to have antedated the neuroleptic era (Bleuler, 1950; Jones and Hunter, 1969), and indeed it has even been suggested that these drugs may actually have contributed to their decline.

3.2.3 *Normal versus abnormal*

Repetitive, often complex, accessory motor activity, which outwardly may appear superfluous, is an integral part of human behaviour and is not merely to be found within the confines of an institution. The social and communicative importance of such activity has been emphasised by those interested in the non-verbal aspects of communication (Argyle, 1972). In the rating of movement disorders, it cannot be assumed that the bounds of 'normality' have already been set in defining the limits of 'dyskinesia' and 'involuntary'. Individual subjects will provide movements to confound even the clearest definitions. Furthermore, the context in which a particular movement pattern occurs may determine its significance. For example, with the wide concept of dyskinesia inherent in the Simpson

Scale, rocking to and fro will require to be evaluated. Rocking, however, can be observed as a response to distress in children and, in certain cultures, as part of the complex social behaviour of grieving. It is not therefore something necessarily confined to patients, and in the context of distress its 'rateable' significance may be diminished.

A clear impression of what is to be considered normal is especially important with the use of standardised, ordinal (ranking) recording schedules. This is because they force a closer examination of the patient than the simple nominal, or present/absent method, the result being higher prevalences. In our own studies, the difference in prevalence between two separate examinations, one using a simple present/absent recording method, the other using the AIMS, was approximately 14%. This was attributable to an increased recognition of 'mild' abnormality when the AIMS was used (Owens *et al.*, 1982). In other words, the closer you look, the more you find. Thus, using rating scales demanding recording on a severity continuum increases the need to be confident in distinguishing mild but pathological movement disorder from non-pathological 'interference'.

Most scales reserve a category ('1') for recording detectable but non-pathological movements. This is in recognition of the fact that with some movements a discrete qualitative change from normal can be difficult to establish, while with others abnormality is no more than a quantitative evaluation. However, a rating of '1' must be used cautiously. Over-reliance on this as a 'not-sure' category will underestimate mild but definite movement disorder. This is particularly important for incidence (rate of onset, as opposed to prevalence) studies or follow-up investigations of early dyskinesia, whose only manifestation may be mild tongue or finger movement (APA Task Force Report, 1979). To ignore definite but minimal dysfunction in these situations would be very misleading.

Certain types of movement should always be considered pathological no matter if present in only mild degree or intermittently. This would apply, for example, to chorea or athetosis/dystonia, though being convinced of the presence of such mild disorder in, say, a tongue which is also tremulous can be difficult. By contrast, rating some types of movement incorporated in a wide range of 'dyskinesia' — such as ankle rotation or finger filliping — is more problematical. A balanced understanding of what is normal and what is not demands a knowledge of the range of movement patterns found in different patient groups, both neurological and psychiatric, as well as a conscious awareness of the variety of motor activity observable in every-day life.

3.2.4 *Factors modifying the clinical signs*
Spontaneous involuntary movement disorders probably have their

pathophysiological basis in disruption of striatal mechanisms (Klawans, 1973a). The movements resulting from this disruption can be modified by a number of non-specific factors whose influence may change the clinical appearance without primarily altering the essential pathophysiological abnormality. Of these, general features of the mental state, especially the affective variable of anxiety-relaxation, are the most important. The more ill at ease the patient, the more prominent the movements are likely to become. Indeed, as with normal people, involuntary activity may only become manifest when the patient is anxious and may disappear in a setting of composure and relaxation.

Few studies systematically consider this type of variable and most ignore it completely. It is, however, important not to disregard the patient's general mental state, particularly when individuals or small groups of subjects are being followed over time. Apparent exacerbations or improvements in spontaneous movements may reflect nothing more than changes in non-specific modifying factors of which general mental state is one of the most relevant, and one for which reliable assessment techniques exist. Features of the mental state cannot be taken for granted, especially, as will be subsequently discussed, in chronic schizophrenic subjects. They have to be sought. It seems a somewhat Pyrrhic endeavour to adhere to standardised examination and rating procedures for involuntary movements, yet omit any assessment (far less a standardised one) of one of their major modifying influences.

Related to anxiety and other features of the mental state is the role of the environment and the amount of stimulation the patient receives. The severity of extrapyramidal movements, especially those subsumed under the heading 'TD', is related to the alertness of the patient. Thus they are at their most intrusive when the subject is aroused and alert, diminish in periods of relaxation and disappear during sleep (APA Task Force Report, 1979). Patients sitting quietly and undisturbed in a chair may betray little that is abnormal, whereas the relatively stimulating context of a formal examination may reveal previously unsuspected involuntary activity. On the other hand, if the patient's attention is actively focused, movements may be partially or completely suppressed, often for quite long periods of time.

The problems of the role of environment are that its components cannot be reliably assessed nor the individual subject's reaction to given surroundings predicted in advance. This is particularly the case with schizophrenic subjects. It is therefore important in baseline prevalence studies with in-patients to carry out the examinations in the patients' own surroundings or, when repeated measures are being contemplated in any subject, that these are conducted in the same surroundings each time. Adopting either an unobtrusive assessment or a formal examination alone, or making evaluations over a brief time interval regardless of the setting, is inadequate to take account of the modifying influence of environment. Assessments, especially in chronic schizophrenics, should combine both a period of observation without the patient's knowledge and a structured formal examination away from distractions, preferably in a room familiar to the subject.

Composure and tranquillity can, of course, be pharmacologically and quite deliberately induced, and have nothing to do with the surroundings. Concurrent drug administration has clear theoretical implications for severity, and possibly prevalence, of movement disorder found at examination (Klawans, 1973b; Casey and Denney, 1977), though in practice the relevance of this remains obscure.

In addition to any specific antidyskinesic activity they may possess, minor tranquillisers such as benzodiazepines produce general sedation which will act to mask spontaneous movement. Furthermore, it has long been known that increasing doses of neuroleptics will, temporarily at least, suppress involuntary motor activity, particularly noted in 'TD' patients, while reduction or cessation of these can lead to a rebound exacerbation (APA Task Force Report, 1979). Sometimes movements are first revealed (or 'released') when neuroleptics are reduced or withdrawn (Gardos *et al.*, 1978). Accurately evaluating non-specific drug effects such as sedation and the probably more receptor-specific neuroleptic effects is, to say the least, a challenge. At a clinical level, one cannot be certain that a prescribed dose of a medication bears any constant relationship to what is actually available to receptor sites. Individual differences in pharmacokinetics and dynamics represent one source of this variability between patients, and although this is a suggested basis for the individual susceptibility of some patients to 'TD' (Jeste *et al.*, 1979), it remains to be proven (Widerlov *et al.*, 1982). However, a far more basic problem within individuals, as well as across groups of patients, relates to the way drugs are often administered, to chronic psychotics in particular, and to their compliance in taking them.

It is known that up to 30% of psychiatric in-patients and as many as 50% of out-patients do not take their medication as recommended — if they take it at all (Willcox *et al.*, 1965). In addition to straightforward non-compliance, some drugs (e.g. anticholinergics, benzodiazepines) may be prescribed with a recommendation that they be taken 'as required'. It is also not uncommon, in the United Kingdom at least, for nurses to exercise considerable discretion in the administration of prescribed medication to in-patients — especially on long-stay wards. Around a baseline, doses may be omitted or additional 'PRN' (i.e. as required) doses given depending on the nursing assessment of the patient's day-to-day requirements.

Trying to relate such unpredictable compliance and flexible administration regimes to the movements detectable on any given day or period of days is an impossible task. This is particularly so if altering the intake of two or more preparations should, in theory produce effects on spontaneous motor activity that are contradictory. For example, according to the dopamine receptor supersensitivity theory of tardive dyskinesia (Klawans, 1973b; Tarsy and Baldessarini, 1977; Marsden and Jenner, 1980), increasing neuroleptic doses should act to suppress involuntary activity, whereas increasing anticholinergics (which might at a routine level be done concomitantly) should act to promote it.

The time sequence for such theoretical events to occur is unknown and we, like others, have not found that neuroleptics *prescribed* at the time of the examination have any significant bearing on the presence of movement disorders when the body is considered as a whole. However, when the detailed Simpson Scale subscores for different body regions are examined separately, those patients being prescribed neuroleptics when seen have a higher prevalence of abnormality in the limbs than those not on neuroleptic prescription. This does not emerge on the AIMS. Thus, some movements included in the wider definitions of dyskinesia (largely but not exclusively tremor) may be more susceptible to modification by concurrent drug prescription and in these circumstances questions of compliance and recommended regimes may be more than theoretical ones. If such issues are relevant, they are likely to be more so in patients whose clinical state is unstable, and in out-patients more than in in-patients.

3.3 Problems inherent in the type of patient

3.3.1 *The schizophrenic as research subject*
Neuroleptics are not only efficacious in the management of acute schizophrenic illnesses (NIMH Collaborative Study Group, 1964). Their long-term (often indefinite) administration is widely advocated to prevent relapse (Leff and Wing, 1971; Hirsch *et al.*, 1973; Davis, 1975). It is in this maintenance role that the risk of neuroleptic-caused dyskinesias would be greatest.

Despite advances in management, it remains the case that a diagnosis of schizophrenia still carries an implication of negative outcome (Harrow *et al.*, 1978). Patients often develop deficits which may subsequently preclude a return to their previous social and occupational level, and indeed may promote their relentless decline. These deficits are widespread, affecting not only their beliefs and experiences but also areas such as cognition and behaviour (Owens and Johnstone, 1980). A characteristic sequela is a volitionless, anhedonic state with restricted ability to express emotion and limited use of verbal communication. This is usually referred to, in the UK at least, as 'the defect state' or more recently as 'negative' schizophrenia, though the end result of an acute schizophrenic illness can include other more 'productive' deficits (Owens and Johnstone, 1980). Post-acute deficits can vary from the barely detectable to the virtually incapacitating, and are to be found both in patients who rely on long-term institutional care as well as in those maintained as outpatients in the community (Owens and Johnstone, 1980; Johnstone et al., 1981). These disabilities cannot therefore be attributed purely to the poverty of the institutional environment in which many chronic patients live.

Schizophrenic patients present unique problems as subjects of objective investigation. This is particularly the case once the chronic deficits of the established illness become manifest. In essence, the examiner has no way of knowing how accurately the features he believes he has elicited reflect the patient's true psychopathology. The patient may not wish to reveal his inner experiences and beliefs or, if mute or thought disordered, may not be able to: he may not understand the questioning or be deliberately evasive: or the abnormalities to which he has fallen victim may be so alien as to defy description in every-day language. One patient said of the experiences inside his head 'It's definitely not thoughts I hear so I suppose it must be a voice — but it's not like any kind of voice I've ever heard before.' The observer has to rely entirely on the patient's own accounts of his inner experiences, from which he must then draw certain inferences. From the research point of view at least, this process forces a qualification on many of our conclusions.

3.3.2 Specific features of the mental state
The relevance of psychic factors of a general kind (e.g. anxiety) to involuntary activity has been noted. In chronic schizophrenics, there are in addition more specific mental-state features that require consideration.

Mental-state abnormalities in chronic schizophrenics are extensive and common (Owens and Johnstone, 1980; Johnstone et al., 1981). The old term, 'burned out', once applied to many long-standing schizophrenics, probably has more relevance in describing the physician's interest than the patients' mental states. Our own studies indicated that only 32 out of 458 chronic in-patients had normal mental states in terms of the assessment procedures used (Owens and Johnstone, 1980).

The features encountered are now often classified into two broad types — 'positive' and 'negative'. While there is little consistency in the literature about what constitutes each of these two groupings of abnormalities, in general it can be said that the former are viewed as phenomena 'added on' to the norm — such as hallucinations, delusions etc. — and the latter are taken to be signs of personality attrition — poverty of speech and restricted or unresponsive affect.

Dysphoric feelings of apprehension or tension can be secondary to psychotic beliefs or experiences which the patient may not manifest behaviourally, far less volunteer in an interview. One well-preserved old gentleman, 50 years in the institution, showed a marked discrepancy in the severity of his movement disorder on two separate occasions. Initially, when his movements were severe, nothing abnormal could be detected in his mental state. It subsequently transpired, however, that he was the discoverer of the secret practice of cosmic poetical psychology which could solve social and industrial strife by the composition of odes. His first assessment coincided with a period of bitter industrial action in the public sector, the solution of which he had been frenetically attempting to bring about by the composition of interminable (and very bad) poems. As the disputes were settled shortly after he had completed a particularly pertinent ode, he felt quite justified in claiming total credit for saving the country from economic chaos, if not civil war — a fact that filled him with contentment. His involuntary movements reflected his satisfaction by being of only moderate severity.

Florid 'positive' features are relatively easily recognised as morbid phenomena and due note can be taken of them. 'Negative' features on the other hand have to be distinguished from such things as resentment, mild parkinsonism and the diffidence of advancing years and social isolation. Their identification is, however, important. We have found that 'negative' features are significantly related to the presence of involuntary movements regardless of age factors and past exposure to neuroleptic drugs, whereas 'positive' features are not (Owens *et al.*, 1983).·Hence the 'negative' clinical picture and involuntary movements may be in some way pathophysiologically related.

The blunted emotional responses characteristic of 'negative' patients act to minimise their observable distress. This does not, however, allow the assumption that because they show no feeling they have none. We have found that 16% of our schizophrenic in-patient sample complained of clinically significant anxiety and/or depression when asked but that this complaint almost always occurred in the context of objective blunting of affect and poverty of speech. These patients felt distressed but did not look it. (Underlying mood disturbance of this sort does not alter the relationship between 'negative' features and spontaneous movements noted above.) Such 'hidden' or purely subjective states may vary over time with little outward alteration in the patient's appearance or behaviour, yet may still act as silent modifying influences on movements, in the same way as do the more conventionally expressed mood states mentioned earlier.

To a large extent it depends on the aims of the study whether or not formal mental-state ratings of such specific features are included. These will, of themselves, present problems, especially with so-called 'negative' states, the assessment of which is of relatively poor reliability. None the less, even if these are not to be formally assessed, it is important to have an awareness of the role they can exercise in modifying the clinical appearance of involuntary movement disorders, especially when carrying out serial evaluations over time.

3.3.3 *Cognitive ability*

In addition to 'positive' and 'negative' mental state features, chronic schizophrenics perform poorly on tests of cognitive ability (Payne, 1973; Owens and Johnstone, 1980). This cognitive impairment has recently been related to CT scan changes suggestive of brain atrophy (Johnstone *et al.*, 1978; Donnelly *et al.*, 1980; Golden *et al.*, 1980) and is unlikely to be merely a phenomenon secondary to inattention, preoccupaton or the like. In general, out-patients are better intellectually preserved than long-stay in-patients (Johnstone *et al.*, 1981) though it is improbable that this is an effect of institutionalisation *per se*. In-patients and out-patients do not significantly differ on other mental state and behavioural variables (Johnstone *et al.*, 1981) and it is possible that suitability for discharge implies, among other things, an ability to perform deductive problem-solving tasks competently.

Many of the neurological conditions associated with the development of spontaneous movements are characterised by intellectual decline to dementia (e.g. Huntington's chorea, Wilson's disease, etc.), and brain damage has often been suggested as a predisposing factor to the development of drug-related movement disorder (Hunter *et al.*, 1964; Crane, 1968). Conflicting results are undoubtedly related to the varying and in general unsatisfactory parameters of brain damage that have been chosen, such as ECT and/or leucotomy. (Although leucotomy can be associated with extensive structural damage (Bydder *et al.*, 1980), the uncomplicated operation is unlikely to give rise to any neurological signs whatsoever — including involuntary movements (Benson *et al.*, 1981).) However, when brain damage is implied from impaired cognitive performance, a relationship with involuntary movements can be established (Edwards, 1970; Owens *et al.*, 1983).

Long-stay schizophrenics vary greatly in their cognitive functioning. Many retain the ability to execute appropriate responses to motor commands, and a number can co-operate with complex instructions. However, overinvolved examination techniques may tax the patient beyond his ability to comprehend and comply. Some of our subjects had difficulty in performing 'activation' procedures that on the face of it were simple. A few left one with the feeling that they could no longer understand what their foot was, far less an instruction to tap it!

Cognitive deficit of such a degree is uncommon and, in particular, is less likely to interfere with examinations in out-patients. None the less, no assumptions can be made regarding the patient's residual cognitive powers, and hence his ability to comply with instructions the examiner may consider elementary. Difficulty in comprehension may promote distress which may raise the level of abnormality above what is truly representative of the patient's deficits.

3.3.4 *The patient's attitude*

This remains one of the 'great unknowns' in evaluating all psychiatric patients, especially if the interviewer is not known to the patient. From what has been said, it is obvious that a subject's misgivings or apprehension regarding an examination will to some extent be reflected in the movement disorder he exhibits. The patient's attitude to examination cannot be predicted or reliably assessed. It is therefore important to assume that *all* subjects are to some extent apprehensive at the outset and to spend the first few minutes of any assessment putting them at their ease. This should perhaps not need to be stated, but the author has seen examiners dive straight into a formal assessment after only the most cursory of introductions — leaving a compliant but bewildered subject. 'Breaking the ice' initially is not just thoughtful. It helps ensure the patient's co-operation and demonstrates a willingness to attempt as thorough and representative an examination as possible. Patients with marked 'negative' deficits coupled with social isolation, especially if they are also institutional residents, are more likely to be unsettled by a formal assessment, as are those who harbour residual persecutory delusions.

A number of rating scales make a recommendation about the duration of the examination. The AIMS, for example, recommends 10 minutes. In theory there is sound reason for this, as it encourages the examiner to allow adequate time for some of the above features to be overcome, hence ensuring that a more representative picture of abnormality is obtained than might be achieved by a cursory approach. As a blanket instruction, however, we did not find this to be helpful in the sort of patients we were dealing with. Apprehension engendered by the mere presence of a stranger was often heightened by over-long examinations, protracted periods of silent observation or over-diligent efforts to elicit a suspected movement by 'activation' or 'reinforcement' techniques, and in some cases this jeopardised the patient's co-operation. (Although all the patients were known to the author over a 3-year period, and all had been examined before, their routine management was the responsibility of other physicians.) We therefore found it necessary to tailor the formal examination to what the patient could be seen to tolerate. With schizophrenics as subjects, pragmatism often has to take precedence over ideals.

3.4 **Problems relating to recording techiques**

3.4.1 *Clinical techniques*
Early publications in the area of movement disorders in neuroleptic-treated subjects were little more than descriptive case reports. Their aim was to highlight what was seen as a new syndrome of (orofacial) involuntary movements. Thus only 'obvious' (i.e. severe) cases were described. When it came to recording prevalence, initial studies were rather impressionistic, and clinicians' differing perception of what was 'obvious' and 'typical' (= severe) was a major factor contributing to the wide discrepancies in the figures that subsequently emerged (from 0.5% to 60%) (Kane and Smith, 1982). (Until comparatively recently, published work often referred to 'incidence' when the subject of investigation was in fact cross-sectional point prevalence, or period prevalence, an error still not uncommon. This illustrates the imprecise use of terminology often employed in clinical psychiatry. There is comparatively little data on the incidence of TD.) In addition heterogeneous diagnostic groups were lumped together. Recently, in line with a general trend towards standardisation in psychiatric research, attempts have been made to improve the reliability of methods for recording spontaneous involuntary motor activity. It is beyond the scope of this chapter to describe the different scales available and only a few comments relevant to the problems of their use will be made.

3.4.1.1 *Examinations.* Most schedules recommend a standard clinical evaluation, combining both an unobtrusive and a formal assessment of all body areas. Most of this chapter has been concerned with some of the many modifying influences that have a bearing on the movements observed in these situations.

Alternatively, some schedules are based on counting techniques (Gardos *et al.*, 1977). The examiner is required to focus on a particular body part and count the movements produced over a stated time interval. This highly objective method offers the prospect of very good inter-rater reliability. However, if too limited a time interval is employed, it runs the very real risk of promoting an unrepresentative impression of the patient's overall abnormality, and short-term fluctuations in clinical pattern or severity will act to compromise test-retest reliability. Furthermore, this method provides a quantitative measure of abnormality and can offer little information on qualitative changes in pattern or distribution within the defined body parts. If they only occur infrequently, it will tend to underestimate the significance of some movements which, it was suggested previously, should always be considered abnormal when present.

Counting methods have been reported to provide satisfactory results but are not as extensively utilised as the basic clinical examination technique.

3.4.1.2 *Recording of findings.*

Rating scales conventionally require findings to be recorded on a numerical scale representing the presence or absence of abnormality and, if present, its severity. The items listed refer to either defined body areas or regions, or individual movements which have been found to be common. Breaking the body up into different parts, or abnormality into particular movements, offers the prospect of providing more detailed information and, by demanding attention to a limited perspective, greater reliability than overall global impressions.

Increasing the complexity of rating scales assumes that it is possible to increase proportionately the examiner's clinical expertise in assessing the individual components of the scale. Such an assumption may not be justified. Crude, rudimentary movements (such as chorea) are irreducible in themselves and cannot be subdivided clinically into component parts. Thus a gross regional or area evaluation of severity is all that is possible. However, for the purposes of completing a formal schedule, movements that retain both their complexity and their co-ordinated relationships may require to be rated on several separate items. Highly detailed schedules such as the Simpson Scale highlight in practice the difficulty of breaking complex co-ordinated motor acts into their constituent parts. Smooth, controlled motor functioning is dependent on a subtle blend of agonist/ antagonist muscle activity, and dissecting this into separate, isolated components is unphysiological. Particular problems arise with orofacial movements to which most scales give greater emphasis. For example, co-ordinated oral activity clearly allows for tongue extrusion to be accompanied by parting of the jaws. Should, therefore, ratings of tongue protrusion automatically be accompanied by ratings of jaw items; or should jaw ratings be reserved purely for movements more intrinsically associated with that area, as for instance grinding or chewing? And if grinding/ chewing alone are the criteria for scoring on jaw items, is concomitant tongue activity that is very likely to accompany these movements to be ignored because it cannot readily be observed?

In practice, difficulties of this type can often be overcome. The point is mentioned to emphasise that further refinement in objective recording in this area may not lie in the production of increasingly lengthy lists comprising more and more detailed movements whose rating may be of doubtful validity. Because features can be elicited with 'acceptable' reliability does not mean that the clinical consensus accurately or meaningfully reflects the pathophysiology — as the history of medicine eloquently demonstrates.

Recommendations are sometimes made (e.g. for the AIMS) that movements which are only elicited with the subject performing some voluntary action in a distant body part ('activation' procedures) be rated one point lower on the severity continuum than movements occurring spontaneously. In the author's experience, movements that emerge only on 'activation' or 'reinforcement' are usually of mild degree — i.e. would in themselves merit a rating of '2'. Applying the above rule would result in contamination of the '1' category, which would then contain movements only elicited during 'activation' but which are none the less considered abnormal as well as movements rated '1' because they are considered not to be abnormal. Applying such a rule seems an unjustified refinement.

3.4.1.3 *Analysis.* Rating scales now conventionally divide the severity continuum on an arbitrary numerical scale with standardised instructions as to what is appropriate to each point (see appendices). In keeping with most scales currently used in clinical psychiatry, the second point on the scale ('1') is allocated to the recording of movements about which the examiner has reservations. Either there is doubt as to whether a particular movement is of abnormal type or else it is not possible to be certain that it is evidenced in sufficient degree to be considered abnormal. Many findings in practice could all too conveniently be rated '1', but the dangers of over-reliance on this have already been emphasised. A further difficulty with this category relates to data analysis.

Data from multi-item rating scales are most conveniently handled by summating the scores on each individual item to a total. Using totals from scales that reserve one point on each item for recording non-pathological or doubtful movements can be misleading, especially if the scale has a large number of items, or if the '1' rating is liberally used. A total score of 4 could clearly result from a single rating of severe degree, and hence of some significance, or from four separate ratings of '1'. Using totals, it is necessary to adopt a cut-off point for normality, which, if it is too low, will inevitably be contaminated by non-pathological '1' ratings. If, on the other hand, it is raised too high, the sensitivity of the data will be compromised by ignoring subjects with mild or moderate, but definitely pathological, movement disorder. A certain amount of contamination either way is inevitable, but will be minimised if the '1' rating is used conservatively and not as an 'anything goes' category.

Rather than using the totals themselves, a global impression can be noted based on an evaluation of the overall abnormality recorded on the individual items. This is useful for classifying patients and makes analysis much easier. However, global impressions are of generally poor reliability and their use greatly reduces the sensitivity of the scale.

As an alternative to totals, analysis can be based on single-symptom criteria — that is, the percentage of the sample achieving a rating of at least 2, 3 or 4, etc. on at least one item. Although this ensures one is only dealing with pathological ratings, it is a limiting method of analysis, as multiple ratings of the same severity are treated as one.

Thus many of the currently available scales present general problems of analysis, especially if they are highly detailed, and no method of retrieving their stored wisdom is entirely satisfactory. In addition analysis of multi-item schedules, the majority of whose components would be expected to receive a 0 rating, presents specific problems which will be referred to elsewhere (see Chapter 7, Section 7.4 and Fig. 7.4).

3.4.2 *Special techniques*

Special techniques using instrumentation to record the presence and severity of involuntary movements offer a degree of objectivity denied to any of the various forms of evaluation by clinicians, and in theory are the ideal. There has been no limit to the ingenuity applied to their development. Refinements of pressure transduction from balloons on the floor of the mouth (Denny and Casey, 1975), or from forces transmitted by the patient 'suspended' on floating platforms, to stress detectors (Korenyi *et al.*, 1974), and ultrasonography (Haines and Sainsbury, 1972) have all been applied.

Unfortunately, the ingenuity behind such techniques has to date usually been inversely proportional to their practicality. They are in general laboratory orientated and require a degree of expertise in their application and in analyses of data. By removing individual judgement they increase reliability, though only if the abnormality elicited during the special circumstances of the assessment is typical. In the author's experience, ultrasonography suffers the major limitation of counting methods in general, in not as yet allowing any qualitative appraisal of the movements it records. For example, it will not adequately distinguish between coarse tremulous movements and mild choreoathetosis. Likewise, any involuntary movements of sufficient degree will be recorded and the examiner still has to be on hand to take account of these. One of the author's patients showed a marked *increase* in recorded movements on an ultrasonic counter after being given a sedative drug, which would seem to negate most of the present chapter. This was, however, due to his 'nodding off'!

Videotape recordings of standardised examinations combine the best of the clinical and special technique approaches. They can be rated subsequent to the examination in a less pressurised atmosphere, by one or more individuals who may, if required, be separate from the examiner involved with the patient. The tape can be re-run as often as required and at different speeds. We have found that twice normal speed can sometimes draw attention to activity overlooked at normal play-back.

The advantages of this precise and, if necessary, permanent record are obvious and the method has been widely advocated (Gardos *et al.*, 1977). Its particular merit is in projects with relatively small numbers of patients where repeated assessments are planned and especially when ratings blind to treatment are involved. Hence the major application of video recording is in therapeutic trials or investigations into the pharmacology of involuntary movements.

The use of video recorders does however have limitations. Especially with institutional patients, they present a strange new situation, the response to which can be unpredictable. Most of our subjects who have been videotaped were surprisingly co-operative but some were unnerved, while others were so absorbed in the technology that their movements diminished noticeably. It is, of course, once again left to the examiner to ensure that a representative record of disability has been taken. Also, in our experience, the two-dimensional picture they provide makes assessment of subtle movements, particularly those of the tongue, very difficult, so the technique may be of less value if the degree of abnormality is slight. In contemplating the use of videotaping, consideration must be given to the enormous investment of time their analysis will demand; accuracy may be achieved at the expense of practicality.

The assessment of involuntary movements has improved considerably in the past decade, though major problems persist. The development of special techniques which are practicable and provide qualitative data is the ideal. However, the objective evaluation of a common and apparently simple involuntary movement like tremor becomes more complex the closer one looks, and it is likely to be some time before the ideal is reached. In the meantime rating scales based on an examiner's assessment will continue to be widely used. It is important to remember that no matter how obsessional the examination, these scales are ordinal (i.e. ranking), not interval (ratio). A rating of 4 implies more abnormality than a rating of 2 — but not twice as much. Ultimately, these scales provide only 'soft' data on trends, recorded numerically to aid statistical evaluation. This should not be used as a justification for decreasing the care given to the assessment of patients, but it does provide a caveat as to conclusions that can be drawn from the ratings.

3.5 Dyskinesia or tardive dyskinesia?

The final dilemma awaiting the researcher in this field, especially in doing prevalence/incidence studies, is what to make of the findings. It must be borne in mind that the term 'dyskinesia' is descriptive whereas adding 'tardive' implies psychotropic drug (particularly neuroleptic) cause. So with what degree of confidence can one imply that the findings obtained reflect drug (neuroleptic) effects or to what extent must such conclusions be qualified because of 'contamination' by other aetiological factors — especially in a schizophrenic population?

All medical diagnosis is based on probability. With some conditions where reliable validating tests are available, it is possible to infer a diagnosis with a high probability of accuracy. Even ignoring the problems which this chapter has highlighted, the differential diagnosis of involuntary movement patterns in chronic schizophrenia is wide and the validating criteria depressingly few. Deciding whether the individual patient is suffering from 'tardive' dyskinesia, spontaneous (idiopathic), orofacial (Altrocchi, 1972) or other dyskinesias (Appenzeller and Biehl, 1968), dyskinesias of senility (Weiner and Klawans, 1973), schizophrenia-related movement disorder (Owens *et al.*, 1982), dyskinesias secondary to oral pathology (Sutcher *et al.*, 1971) or any one of the many conditions involved in the differential diagnosis of choreoathetosis (Granacher, 1981) can be a daunting task. Yet the implications of these diagnoses are different, so it is important to attempt their separation.

It might be reasonable to suppose, going back to Uhrbrand and Faurbye's (1960) original concept of 'neuroleptic-caused' dyskinesia, that the presence of a history of exposure to neuroleptic drugs would be adequate to validate the diagnosis of 'tardive' dyskinesia. In our own work, however, we could not show this to be the case. We could not identify any notable differences in the prevalence, severity and distribution of involuntary movements between chronic schizophrenics simply on the basis of the presence or absence of a history of neuroleptic exposure (Owens *et al.*, 1982).

The fact is that neuroleptic drugs are neither necessary nor sufficient to account for the development of involuntary movement disorders. Similar clinical abnormalities to those found in 'tardive dyskinesia' can occur in patients never exposed to psychotropic medication, and taken overall probably only a minority of schizophrenics on long-term maintenance treatment develop abnormal movements. Other variables, such as age, length of illness, factors directly associated with the illness itself and factors of individual susceptibility are also of relevance. Until the contribution of all of these can be evaluated, implications of cause in individual cases cannot be made with high levels of confidence.

This chapter has attempted to illustrate a general point using one specific example, though from the field of clinical research many could have been chosen. In psychiatry, it is hardly possible to be aware of, far less account for, all the potential factors that come to bear on a given question, and many interposing, non-specific variables will modify clinical findings. It behoves investigators to pay meticulous attention to those factors that can be evaluated and controlled, and to foster a healthy criticism of results based on appreciation of the general influences that may have remained beyond their control.

References

Altrocchi, P.H. (1972). Spontaneous oral-facial dyskinesia. *Arch. Neurol.* **26**, 506–12.

American Psychiatric Association Task Force on late neurological effects of antipsychotic drugs (1979). Tardive Dyskinesia. American Psychiatric Association, Washington DC. (Also summerised (1980), *Am. J. Psychiat.* **137**, 1163–72.)

Appenzeller, O. and Biehl, J.P. (1968). Mouthing in the elderly: a cerebellar sign. *J. Neurol. Sci.* **6**, 249–60.

Argyle, M. (1972). Non-verbal communication in human social interaction. In *Non-verbal Communication* (R.A. Hinde, Ed.), Cambridge University Press, Cambridge.

Ayd, Jr F.J. (1961). A survey of drug-induced extrapyramidal reactions. *J. Amer. Med. Assoc.,* **175**, 1054–60.

Benson, D.F., Stuss, D.T., Naeser, M.A., Weir, W.S., Kaplan, E.F. and Levine, H.L. (1981). The long-term effects of prefrontal leucotomy. *Arch. Neurol.* **38**, 165–9.

Bleuler, E. (1950). *Dementia Praecox or the Group of Schizophrenias*, International Universities Press, New York.

Boice, R. and Kraemer, E.A. (1981) Stereotypies as behavioural indices in mental patients. *J. Non-verbal Behav.* **6**, 30–45.

Bydder, G.A., Kreel, L., Owens, D.G. C. and Johnstone, E.C. (1980). Computed tomography after leucotomy. *J. Comput. Tomography* **4**, 43–7.

Casey, D.E. and Denney, D. (1977). Pharmacological characterisation of tardive dyskinesia. *Psychopharmacology* **54**, 1–8.

Crane, G.E. (1968). Tardive dyskinesia in patients treated with major neuroleptics. *Amer. J. Psychiat.* **124** (Feb. suppl.), 40–8.

Crane, G.E. and Naranjo, E.R., (1971). Motor disorders induced by neuroleptics. *Arch. Gen. Psychiat.* **24**, 179–84.

Crow, T.J., Cross, A.J., Johnstone, E.C., Owen, F., Owens, D.G.C. and Waddington, J.L. (1981). Tardive dyskinesia — disease process or drug effect? In *Biological Psychiatry (Proceedings of IIIrd World Congress of Biological Psychiatry)* (C. Perris, G. Struwe and B. Jansson, Eds), Elsevier/North Holland.

Davis, J.M. (1975). Overview: maintenance Therapy in Psychiatry: I. Schizophrenia. *Amer. J. Psychiat.* **132**, 1237–45.

Denny, D. and Casey, D. (1975). An objective method for measuring dyskinetic movements in tardive dyskinesia. *Electroencephal. Clin. Neurophysiol.* **38**, 645–6.

Donnelly, E.F., Weinberger, D.R., Waldman, I.N. and Wyatt, R.J. (1980). Cognitive impairment associated with morphological brain abnormalities on computed tomography in chronic schizophrenic patients. *J. Nerv. Ment. Dis.* **168**, 305–8.

Edwards, H. (1970). The significance of brain damage in persistent oral dyskinesia. *Brit. J. Psychiat.* **116**, 271–5.

Faurbye, A., Rasch, P-J., Bender-Petersen, P., Brandberg, G. and Pakkenberg,

H. (1964). Neurological symptoms in pharmacotherapy of psychoses. *Acta Psychiat. Scand.* **40**, 10–27.

Gardos, G., Cole, J.O. and La Brie, R. (1977). The assessment of tardive dyskinesia. *Arch. Gen. Psychiat.* **34**, 1206–12.

Gardos, G., Cole, J.O. and Tarsy, D. (1978). Withdrawal syndromes associated with antipsychotic drugs. *Amer. J. Psychiat.* **135**, 1321–4.

Golden, C.J., Moses, J.A., Zelazowski, R., Graber, B., Zata, L.M., Horvath, T.B. and Berger, P.A. (1980). Cerebral ventricular size and neuropsychological impairment in young chronic schizophrenics. *Arch. Gen. Psychiat.* **37**, 619–23.

Granacher, Jr. R.P. (1981). Differential diagnosis of tardive dyskinesia: an overview. *Amer. J. Psychiat.* **138**, 1288–97.

Guy, W. (1976). ECDEU Assessment Manual for Psychopharmacology. Department of Health, Education and Welfare, Washington, D.C. pp. 534–7.

Haines, J. and Sainsbury, P. (1972) Ultrasound system for measuring patient's activity and disorders of movement. *Lancet* **ii**, 802–3.

Hall, R.A., Jackson, R.B. and Swain, J.M. (1956) Neurotoxic reactions resulting from chlorpromazine administration. *J. Amer. Med. Assoc.* **161**, 214–18.

Harrow, M., Grinker, P.R., Silverstein, M.L. and Holzman, P. (1978). Is modern-day schizophrenic outcome still negative? *Amer. J. Psychiat.* **135**, 1156–62.

Hirsch, S.R., Gaind, R., Rohde, P.D., Stevens, B.C. and Wing, J.K. (1973). Out-patient maintenance of chronic schizophrenic patients with long-acting fluphenazine: double-blind placebo trial. *Brit. Med. J.* **1**, 633–7.

Hunter, R., Earl, C.J. and Janz, D. (1964). A syndrome of abnormal movements and dementia in leucotomised patients treated with phenothiazines. *J. Neurol. Neurosurg. Psychiat.* **27**, 219–23.

Jeste, D.V., Rosenblatt, J.E., Wagner, R.L. and Wyatt, R.J. (1979). High serum neuroleptic levels in tardive dyskinesia? *New Engl. J. Med.* **301**, 1184.

Jeste, D.V. and Wyatt, R.J. (1981). Changing epidemiology of tardive dyskinesia: an overview. *Amer. J. Psychiat.* **138**, 297–309.

Johnstone, E.C., Crow, T.J., Frith, C.D., Stevens, M., Kreel, L. and Husband, J. (1978). The dementia of dementia praecox. *Acta Psychiat. Scand.* **57**, 305–24.

Johnstone, E.C., Owens, D.G C., Gold, A., Crow, T.J. and Macmillan, J.F. (1981). Institutionalisation and the defects of schizophrenia. *Brit. J. Psychiat.* **139**, 195–203.

Jones, M. and Hunter, R. (1969). Abnormal movements in patients with chronic psychiatric illness. In *Psychotropic Drugs and Dysfunctions of the Basal Ganglia. Proceedings of Workshop at Bethesda, MD* (G.E. Crane and J. Gardner, Eds), Public Health Service Publication, No. 1938, NIMH, Bethesda, MD.

Kane, J.M. and Smith, J.M. (1982). Tardive dyskinesia. Prevalence and risk factors 1959–1979. *Arch. Gen. Psychiat.* **39**, 473–81.

Klawans, H.L. (1973a). *The Pharmacology of Extrapyramidal Movement Disorders*, S. Karger, Basel.

Klawans, H.L. (1973b). The pharmacology of tardive dyskinesias. *Amer. J. Psychiat.* **130**, 82–6.

Korenyi, C., Whittier, J.R. and Fischbach, G. (1974). Cineseismography: a method for measuring abnormal involuntary movements of the human body. *Dis. Nerv. Syst.* **35**, 63–5.

Kramer, D.A. and McKinney, W.T. (1979). The overlapping territories of psychiatry and ethology. *J. Nerv. Ment. Dis.* **167**, 3–22.

Leff, J.P. and Wing, J.K. (1971). Trial of maintenance therapy in schizophrenia. *Brit. Med. J.* **2**, 599–604.

Marsden, C.D. and Jenner, P. (1980). The pathophysiology of extrapyramidal side-effects of neuroleptic drugs. *Psychol. Med.* **10**, 55–72.

Marsden, C.D., Tarsy, D. and Baldessarini, R.J. (1975). Spontaneous and drug-induced movement disorders in psychotic patients. In *Psychiatric Aspects of Neurological Disease* (D.F. Benson and D. Blumer, Eds), Grune & Stratton, New York.

Melvin, K.E.W. (1962). Tetanus-like reactions to the phenothiazine drugs. 'The Grimacing Syndrome'. *New Zealand Med. J.* **61**, 90–2

National Institute of Mental Health Psychopharmacology Service Centre Collaborative Study Group (1964). Phenothiazine treatment in acute schizophrenia. *Arch. Gen. Psychiat.* **10**, 246–61.

Owens, D.G.C. and Johnstone, E.C. (1980). The disabilities of chronic schizophrenia — their nature and factors contributing to their development. *Brit. J. Psychiat.* **136**, 384–95.

Owens, D.G.C., Johnstone, E.C. and Frith, C.D. (1982). Spontaneous involuntary disorders of movement: their prevalence, severity and distribution in chronic schizophrenics with and without treatment with neuroleptics. *Arch. Gen. Psychiat.* **39**, 452–61.

Owens, D.G.C., Johnstone, E.C. and Frith, C.D. (1983). Factors associated with the presence of involuntary movements in chronic schizophrenic in-patients. Abstracts of VIIth World Congress of Psychiatry, 11–16 July 1983, Vienna.

Paulson, G.W. (1981). Treatment of tardive dyskinesia. In *Disorders of Movement* (A. Barbeau, Ed.), MTP Press, Lancaster.

Payne, R.W. (1973). Cognitive abnormalities. In *The Handbook of Abnormal Psychology* (H.J. Eysenck, Ed.), Pitman, London.

Randrup, A. and Munkvad, I. (1967). Stereotyped activities produced by amphetamine in several animal species and man. *Psychopharmacologia* **11**, 300–10.

Simpson, G.M., Lee, J.H., Zoubok, B. and Gardos, G. (1979). A rating scale for tardive dyskinesia. *Psychopharmacology* **64**, 171–9.

Sutcher, H.D., Underwood, R.B., Beatty, R.A. and Sugar, O. (1971). Orofacial dyskinesia: a dental dimension. *J. Amer. Med. Assoc.* **216**, 1459–63.

Tarsy, D. and Baldessarini, R.J. (1977). The pathophysiologic basis of tardive dyskinesia. *Biol. Psychiat.* **12**, 431–50.

Turek, I.S. (1975). Drug-induced dyskinesia: reality or myth? *Dis. Nerv. Syst.* **36**, 397–9.

Uhrbrand, L. and Faurbye, A. (1960). Reversible and irreversible dyskinesia after treatment with perphenazine, chlorpromazine, reserpine and electroconvulsive therapy. *Psychopharmacologia* **1**, 408–18.

Weiner, W.J. and Klawans, H.L. (1973). Lingual–facial–buccal movements in the elderly. *J. Amer. Geriat. Soc.* **21**, 314–20.

Widerlov, E., Haggstrom, J-E., Kilts, C.D., Anderson, U., Breese, G.R. and Mailman, R.B. (1982). Serum concentrations of thioridazine, its major metabolites, and serum neuroleptic-like activities in schizophrenics with and without tardive dyskinesia. *Acta Psychiat. Scand.* **66**, 294–305.

Willcox, D.R.C., Gillan, R. and Hare, E.H. (1965). Do psychiatric out-patients take their drugs? *Brit. Med. J.* **2**, 790–2.

Appendix 3.1

ABNORMAL INVOLUNTARY MOVEMENT SCALE (AIMS)

	STUDY	PATIENT	FORM	PERIOD	RATER	HOSPITAL
			117			
	(1.6)	(7.9)	(10.12)	(13.15)	(16.17)	(79.80)

PATIENT'S NAME

RATER

DATE

INSTRUCTIONS:	Complete Examination Procedure (reverse side) before making ratings. MOVEMENT RATINGS: Rate highest severity observed. Rate movements that occur upon activation one *less* than those observed spontaneously.	Code:	0 = None 1 = Minimal, may be extreme normal 2 = Mild 3 = Moderate 4 = Severe

		(Circle One)	CARD 01 (18.19)
FACIAL AND ORAL MOVEMENTS:	1. **Muscles of Facial Expression** e.g., movements of forehead, eyebrows, periorbital area, cheeks; include frowning, blinking, smiling, grimacing	0 1 2 3 4	(20)
	2. **Lips and Perioral Area** e.g., puckering, pouting, smacking	0 1 2 3 4	(21)
	3. **Jaw** e.g., biting, clenching, chewing, mouth opening, lateral movement	0 1 2 3 4	(22)
	4. **Tongue** Rate only increase in movement both in and out of mouth, NOT inability to sustain movement	0 1 2 3 4	(23)

Category	#	Item	Ratings					Code
EXTREMITY MOVEMENTS:	5.	**Upper** (*arms, wrists, hands, fingers*) Include choreic movements, (i.e., rapid, objectively purposeless, irregular, spontaneous), athetoid movements (i.e., slow, irregular, complex, serpentine). Do NOT include tremor (i.e., repetitive, regular, rhythmic)	0	1	2	3	4	(24)
	6.	**Lower** (*legs, knees, ankles, toes*) e.g., lateral knee movement, foot tapping, heel dropping, foot squirming, inversion and eversion of foot	0	1	2	3	4	(25)
TRUNK MOVEMENTS:	7.	**Neck, shoulders, hips** e.g., rocking, twisting, squirming, pelvic gyrations	0	1	2	3	4	(26)
	8.	Severity of abnormal movements	None, normal — 0 / Minimal — 1 / Mild — 2 / Moderate — 3 / Severe — 4					(27)
GLOBAL JUDGMENTS:	9.	Incapacitation due to abnormal movements	None, normal — 0 / Minimal — 1 / Mild — 2 / Moderate — 3 / Severe — 4					(28)
	10.	Patient's awareness of abnormal movements Rate only patient's report	No awareness — 0 / Aware, no distress — 1 / Aware, mild distress — 2 / Aware, moderate distress — 3 / Aware, severe distress — 4					(29)
DENTAL STATUS:	11.	Current problems with teeth and/or dentures	No — 0 / Yes — 1					(30)
	12.	Does patient usually wear dentures?	No — 0 / yes — 1					(31)

Appendix 3.1 *continued*   Examination Procedure

Either before or after completing the Examination Procedure observe the patient unobtrusively, at rest (e.g., in waiting room).

The chair to be used in this examination should be a hard, firm one without arms.

1. Ask patient whether there is anything in his/her mouth (i.e., gum, candy, etc.) and if there is, to remove it.

2. Ask patient about the *current* condition of his/her teeth. Ask patient if he/she wears dentures. Do teeth or dentures bother patient *now*?

3. Ask patient whether he/she notices any movements in mouth, face, hands, or feet. If yes, ask to describe and to what extent they *currently* bother patient or interfere with his/her activities.

4. Have patient sit in chair with hands on knees, legs slightly apart, and feet flat on floor. (Look at entire body for movements while in this position).

5. Ask patient to sit with hands hanging unsupported. If male, between legs, if female and wearing a dress, hanging over knees. (Observe hands and other body areas.)

6. Ask patient to open mouth. (Observe tongue at rest within mouth.) Do this twice.

7. Ask patient to protrude tongue. (Observe abnormalities of tongue movement.) Do this twice.

8. Ask patient to tap thumb, with each finger, as rapidly as possible for 10–15 seconds; separately with right hand, then with left hand. (Observe facial and leg movements.)

9. Flex and extend patient's left and right arms (one at a time.) (Note any rigidity and rate on DOTES.)

10. Ask patient to stand up. (Observe in profile. Observe all body areas again, hips included.)

*11. Ask patient to extend both arms outstretched in front with palms down. (Observe trunk, legs, and mouth.)

*12. Have patient walk a few paces, turn, and walk back to chair. (Observe hands and gait.) Do this twice.

* Activated movements

Appendix 3.2 Rockland Research Institute: Tardive dyskinesia rating scale (Simpson *et al.*, 1979)

Patient _____ _____ 1 a.m.
Date _____ Time_____ p.m.
Setting _____ Rather_____

Absent

?

Mild

Moderate

Moderately severe

Very severe

		Absent	?	Mild	Moderate	Moderately severe	Very severe
FACE							
1.	Blinking of eyes	0	1	2	3	4	5
2.	Tremor of eyelids	0	1	2	3	4	5
3.	Tremor of upper lip (rabbit syndrome)	0	1	2	3	4	5
4.	Pouting of the (lower) lip	0	1	2	3	4	5
5.	Puckering of lips	0	1	2	3	4	5
6.	Sucking movements	0	1	2	3	4	5
7.	Chewing movements	0	1	2	3	4	5
8.	Smacking of lips	0	1	2	3	4	5
9.	Bon-bon sign	0	1	2	3	4	5
10.	Tongue protrusion	0	1	2	3	4	5
11.	Tongue tremor	0	1	2	3	4	5
12.	Choreoathetoid movements of the tongue	0	1	2	3	4	5
13.	Facial tics	0	1	2	3	4	5
14.	Grimacing	0	1	2	3	4	5
15.	Other (describe) _____	0	1	2	3	4	5
16.	Other (describe) _____	0	1	2	3	4	5
NECK AND TRUNK							
17.	Head nodding	0	1	2	3	4	5
18.	Retrocollis	0	1	2	3	4	5
19.	Spasmodic torticollis	0	1	2	3	4	5
20.	Torsion movements (trunk)	0	1	2	3	4	5
21.	Axial hyperkinesia	0	1	2	3	4	5
22.	Rocking movement	0	1	2	3	4	5
23.	Other (describe) _____	0	1	2	3	4	5
24.	Other (describe) _____	0	1	2	3	4	5

Appendix 3.2 (*continued*)

	Absent	?	Mild	Moderate	Moderately severe	Very severe

EXTREMITIES (Upper)

25. Ballistic movements	0	1	2	3	4	5
26. Choreoathetoid movements — fingers	0	1	2	3	4	5
27. Choreoathetoid movements — wrists	0	1	2	3	4	5
28. Pill-rolling movements	0	1	2	3	4	5
29. Caressing or rubbing face and hair	0	1	2	3	4	5
30. Rubbing of thighs	0	1	2	3	4	5
31. Other (describe) _____	0	1	2	3	4	5
32. Other (describe) _____	0	1	2	3	4	5

(Lower)

33. Rotation and/or flexion of ankles	0	1	2	3	4	5
34. Toe movements	0	1	2	3	4	5
35. Stamping movements — standing	0	1	2	3	4	5
36. Stamping movement — sitting	0	1	2	3	4	5
37. Restless legs	0	1	2	3	4	5
38. Crossing/uncrossing legs — sitting	0	1	2	3	4	5
39. Other (describe) _____	0	1	2	3	4	5
40. Other (describe) _____	0	1	2	3	4	5

ENTIRE BODY

41. Holokinetic movements	0	1	2	3	4	5
42. Akathisia	0	1	2	3	4	5
43. Other (describe) _____	0	1	2	3	4	5

COMMENTS

_____

_____

_____

4 *Michael H. Joseph, Raymond Lofthouse*
Stephen J. Gamble and John L. Waddington

Sampling of tissues and body fluids

4.1 Introduction

In the collection of animal tissues and fluids the immediate requirement is fixation to stop biochemical processes within them which may lead to changes in the substances to be measured.

For certain purposes, e.g. enzyme determination, studies on intact cells or subcellular fractions, it may not be permissible to freeze the tissue. In such a case, rapid homogenisation in an ice-cold medium is required, followed by immediate analysis.

The analyses described in Chapters 5 and 6 can be carried out on frozen tissue, and thus samples can be frozen as obtained, stored at suitable temperatures (-20 to $-170°C$) and analysed in batches. This also has the advantage that most metabolites and enzymes are more stable in the undisrupted tissue, and that additional assays can subsequently be carried out on frozen samples, whereas homogenates would be less versatile. If assays are to be carried out at different times, it is important to dice and mix the tissue before storage.

The analyses in Chapters 5 and 6 do not require particularly rapid fixation. If this is required, for instance for the measurement of rapidly cycling high-energy intermediates or acetylcholine, then special techniques such as microwave irradiation (heat fixation), immersion in liquid nitrogen or freeze blowing must be used (see also Rodnight, 1975). Fixation of rat tissues by freezing following removal at ambient temperatures and dissection at $4°C$ will be described in section 4.2. Tissue from primates (other than humans) is dealt with in Chapter 2, section 5. Additional considerations for human tissue will be covered in the final section of this chapter.

4.2 Rat tissue

4.2.1 *Brain*
The rat brain is most easily removed from the head after decapitation. For most biochemical studies rats are stunned by a blow on the head, but for study of the brain, the blow should be directed to the back of the neck or the thorax. In the latter case the heart will usually be stopped, and this technique is therefore not suitable where blood is also to be collected. If blood is required, a small animal guillotine such as the Harvard CN 130 can be used. Animals can be lightly anaesthetised with ether or a barbiturate but the anaesthetic agent may itself have confounding neurochemical effects. Decapitation of of the conscious animal in the guillotine is perfectly humane in the hands of a practised operator. The collection of blood is detailed in section 4.2.3.

For brain removal after decapitation, the skin overlying the skull is cut along the midline, most easily from the rear, and dissected back to expose the dorsal skull plates which should be scraped free of adhering material (periosteum). It is then useful to split the skull plates along the midline by introducing the points of a pair of strong scissors or bone-cutters above and below the dorsal skull at the exposed (trunk) end, followed by a cutting and twisting movement. Particular care is needed if cerebellar and brainstem tissue are required. It is important to note that the level of decapitation in the anterior–posterior (front-back) direction should be selected with regard to the tissue required. The more anterior the level, the more easily the removal of the forebrain can be effected; however, such a level of decapitation may leave cerebellar and brainstem tissue with the trunk. Having split the dorsal skull plates, these can be (carefully) removed with twisting movements of strong forceps, to expose the underlying brain. Skull should be removed to a sufficient width to allow unimpeded exit of the brain from its cavity. If not removed with overlying skull, the lining of the brain (dura) must be removed also. It can be dissected by introducing the point of small scissors or forceps along the midline and cutting/pulling free. The brain is most easily removed by raising the skull, by the snout, to an angle of 45–90° from the horizontal and introducing the end of a spatula or the closed ends of a pair of forceps down at the very front of the brain, severing the olfactory bulbs; gently pulling back will then ease the brain from its cavity subject to cutting the optic nerves near the chiasma. Removal of cerebellum and brainstem with the forebrain will require careful splitting of bone at the trunk end of the head to allow unimpeded exit. For removal of the forebrain with olfactory bulbs intact, careful frontal excavation with bone-cutters is required.

Once removed, selection of an appropriate procedure for brain dissection is influenced by the region to be studied and the stability of the material to be assayed therein. For the gross cerebral regions (e.g. cortex, striatum, hippocampus, thalamus, hypothalamus, cerebellum, brainstem, etc.), the brain can be placed freshly on a glass plate set in ice and subjected to blunt dissection with forceps according to a standard technique (e.g. Glowinski and Iversen, 1966). We have evolved what we consider to be a useful variant of this coarse blunt dissection of the forebrain, in which we proceed as follows. The closed tips of curved forceps (fine points) are introduced along and down into the dorsal midline of the brain. Pressure is then released so that the natural 'spring' in the forceps parts the cortices of the two hemispheres down to just below the level of the corpus callosum (appearing as a thin, white band under the dorsal cortex). The cortices are then gently 'peeled' sideways to expose the striatum of each hemisphere. The medial extents of the striata are then carefully separated from the central midbrain portion. From this preparation, the exposed striata and hippocampi can be 'pinched' out by use of the same forceps. The 'wings' of the two cortices can then be separated from the midbrain portion also. By inverting this residual tissue, the hypothalamus can be cut free by running a very fine pointed scalpel blade round the hypothalamic area to a depth of a couple of millimetres and pinching free. The principal residual tissue is now thalamus which can be freed from other regional contaminants by careful blunt dissection. As always, careful and repeated practice is the secret of achieving a rapid coarse dissection with the minimum of contamination of tissue.

The dissection of more discrete areas is influenced by the extent to which contamination by surrounding tissue can be tolerated; small areas such as the nucleus accumbens can be blunt-dissected from fresh tissue, with some risk of possible contamination as in the procedure of Horn *et al.* (1974). However, for greater accuracy the brain can be quickly frozen, and thick (0.5–2 mm) sections cut on a freezing microtome; the required regions can then be dissected from such sections on the microtome stage using a fine scalpel blade (Waddington and Cross, 1978). Use of an electronic freezing unit with continuously variable stage temperature (e.g. that supplied by Mectron (Frigistor) Ltd) will allow rapid control of optimum temperatures for attachment of brain and section to the stage and for dissection; dissection from too cold a section may result in a carefully dissected sample chipping or flying off the stage to be contaminated on the bench or lost on the laboratory floor. For very fine microdissection, such as individual thalamic or hypothalamic nuclei, the use of a fine-bore tissue punch and much thinner frozen sections, perhaps aided by a dissecting microscope, may be required (Palkovits 1973).

The brain samples are placed in tubes of a suitable size and frozen in a freezing misture (acetone or methanol/dry ice) before storage; we use a deep freeze at −40°C for general purposes. Alternatively tubes precooled in pelleted dry ice can be used and replaced in the pelleted dry ice. It is important to use tubes with a securely sealing top (seal must be good at −40°C also) and ones that are not too large for the samples so as to avoid tissue drying out or taking up water in the freezer, for the reasons given in Chapter 5.

4.2.2 *Cerebrospinal fluid*

The rat is not of course the ideal animal for CSF studies, and larger animals such as rabbits are frequently used. Nonetheless the abundance of biochemical, pharmacological and psychological information available on the rat does lead to a requirement for CSF on occasion.

CSF can be taken from the terminally anaesthetised rat by flexing the animal's neck over an angled support. The skin and neck muscles are incised and the membrane (creamy coloured) covering the cisternum between the base of the skull and the first vertebra is pierced with a short fine needle on a 1 ml syringe. Up to 200 μl of CSF can be obtained from a 300 g rat.

Small samples (< 100 μl) can be obtained repetitively from rats *in vivo* by chronically implanting a guide tube with a self-sealing stopper along the back of the skull, with its end resting on the membrane (Kiser, 1982). In animals accustomed to the procedure, samples can be taken from the conscious animal; a cannula needle slightly longer than the guide tube is used.

4.2.3 *Blood*

Reasonable quantities of rat blood can be obtained from the trunk following sacrifice by decapitation of the conscious animal. The spout of a large polythene funnel is cut at right angles so that its inside diameter is just less than the outside diameter of a blood collection tube (Fig. 4.1). The inside of the funnel is wetted with heparin (rat blood clots extremely readily); the blood collection tube is inserted and pulled almost through the funnel. The tube is placed in a rack near to the guillotine, the animal's trunk is grasped firmly with the non-preferred hand, and the animal is decapitated. The trunk is immediately held firmly neck down into the funnel using the same hand. Between 5 and 10 ml of blood is collected from a 200 g rat. The tube is removed downwards from the funnel, capped, gently inverted several times and placed in an ice bucket.

Samples of whole blood can be snap frozen before storage as described in Chapter 5. Plasma is obtained by centrifugation of whole blood at ~2000 g for 10 min at ~4°C.

Larger amounts of blood per animal can be obtained under terminal nembutal anaesthesia by opening the peritoneal cavity and inserting a fine needle into the abdominal aorta, or a large needle through the diaphragm

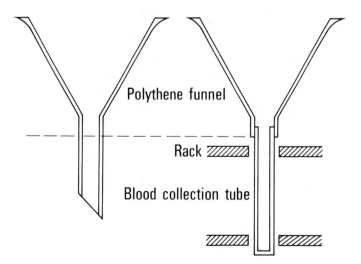

Fig. 4.1. Rat trunk blood collection device.

into the heart. For collection of rat platelets this procedure will give a much better yield. The syringe used to draw blood should contain an appropriate volume of ACD (section 4.3.3) and after separating platelets by differential centrifugation, as described for human blood, a wash in 1% ammonium oxalate will selectively lyse red cells leaving a good yield of platelets.

4.3 **Human tissue**

4.3.1 *Human post-mortem brain tissue*
4.3.1.1 *Legal requirements.* The removal of human tissue at post-mortem examination and its subsequent use is subject, in the United Kingdom, to the provisions of the Human Tissues Act (HMSO, 1961). Under this act permission has either to have been granted by the deceased prior to death or to be granted after death by the person lawfully in charge of the body. In those cases where a coroner is involved his consent must also be obtained.

4.3.1.2 *Safety requirements.* In the United Kingdom unfixed human brain and spinal cord material is classified in the Howie Report (Howie, 1978) as requiring at least category B2 conditions of containment and in certain situations the stricter B1 conditions. The procedures and precautions outlined for these categories should be strictly adhered to at all times when handling this material. At the post mortem it is advisable that a 2–5 ml sample of blood should be collected to be tested before dissection of the brain for Australia antigen (also known at hepatitis B surface antigen [HBsAg]) to exclude the possibility of infection by serum hepatitis virus.

The safety requirements outlined in the Howie Report should be borne in mind at all times when handling biological tissues and physiological fluids, both human and animal, and any work carried out on brain tissue which is likely to generate splashing or produce aerosols should be carried out inside a suitable biological safety cabinet. The design of the cabinet and its installation should be in accordance with established standards (e.g. BS 5726: British Standards Institution, 1979). Guidelines on the siting and installation of biological safety cabinets are detailed in Monograph 6 of the Public Health Laboratory Service (Collins *et al.*, 1974).

4.3.1.3 *Collection and documentation.* Active co-operation between the investigator, coroner, hospital and mortuary staff is essential to ensure that the body is transferred as rapidly as possible after death to the mortuary refrigerator and that notification is given of post-mortem times and arrangements. These factors are important to ensure that freezing of the brain can take place as soon as possible after its removal from the body in order to minimise, and control for, time-dependent effects on biochemical and other parameters (Cross and Owen, 1979). It is a good policy to obtain maximum information about the patient at the time of collection as later contact with the hospital and access to patient records can be difficult. The important information includes patient name, sex, age, weight, hospital, hospital number, diagnosis, regular medication and drugs administered up to death, cause of death, date and time of death, time when body was refrigerated, and date and time of post mortem. We have found that a standard duplicated form is the most effective means of recording these details. Subsequently this data may be transferred to a computer database (see Chapter 7 on record keeping and data analysis).

In order to preserve the natural brain shape and facilitate later dissection we have fashioned polystyrene moulds into which, after lining with polythene or 'cling-film', the brain is inverted for freezing. The moulds are fashioned using a two-part foam mix (Strand Glass Fibre Ltd, Brentway Trading Estate, Brentford, Middlesex, England) and a plaster cast taken from the inside of the cranial vault of a human skull. Once frozen, the brain can be easily removed from the mould (which is reusable) and stored in double plastic bags at $-40°C$ to $-70°C$.

4.3.1.4 *Dissection and storage.* This is carried out within a Class I Microbiological Cabinet as defined by British Standard 5726 (British Standards Institution, 1979). The brain, after being allowed to slightly thaw and soften, is placed on a white perspex plate sitting either on an electrical cooling tray or, as we currently use, a plastic tray containing dry ice (solid carbon dioxide) pellets. The brain is sliced, using a brain knife, into serial coronal sections (approximately 3 mm thick) and these are laid out sequentially. Dissection of the various areas can then be carried out in conjunction with a suitable brain atlas (e.g. De Armond *et al.*, 1974). It is very important that consistency be maintained between dissections, particularly where more than one person is involved. The demarcation of areas should be closely defined especially for those which are less easily identifiable. Differences in results reported by different groups of workers have been attributed to their dissection techniques (Bird *et al.*, 1979; Crow *et al.*, 1980).

Once an area has been dissected out from adjacent sections the pieces should be chopped and mixed together to provide a homogeneous sample. It can now be stored, preferably over liquid nitrogen, in suitable tubes or containers (e.g. screw-topped, 2 ml vials — Nunc Cryotube N1076-1A) adequately labelled. A record of the areas dissected from each brain should be added to the file. If possible, a note should also be made on the file of the dates on which a part of any sample is removed for analysis.

4.3.2 *Human cerebrospinal fluid*

Human CSF is usually obtained by lumbar puncture. This procedure is reviewed by Patten (1977) and by Simpson (1980). CSF for research purpose is obtained as that surplus to clinical and diagnostic requirements, or in its own right after the necessary ethical permission has been obtained. Routine centrifugation of CSF is useful to remove cellular material. Ventricular CSF can also be collected directly from the brain at post mortem.

The conditions of storage can be critical for CSF. For example Tyrrell *et al.* (1979) have shown that the cytopathic effect observed in tissue culture cells in some CSF samples is lost after a few weeks' storage at $-40°C$ but is preserved for long periods at $-70°C$ or if the samples are stored over liquid nitrogen.

Aliquots of the collected material are stored in suitable sterile screw-topped containers (e.g. Nunc tubes as above) in a liquid nitrogen refrigerator, if possible without further preservative.

The antibiotic Bacitracin (Sigma, Poole, England), at a final concentration of 0.45 mM is used as an inhibitor of peptide degradation in samples required for peptide estimation. These samples should be stored as cold as possible. Ascorbate is often added as an antioxidant for amine metabolites, but may lead to problems if HPLC–EC is used. In general, rapid freezing gives more flexibility and is preferable to preservatives, unless the latter are positively indicated.

4.3.3 *Human blood fractions*

4.3.3.1 *Collection and safety requirements.* Blood is collected by venepuncture, usually from an antecubital vein, gently transferred into suitable tubes (BS 4851; British Standards Institution, 1975) and gently mixed by inversion or rotation. Samples can be taken at this stage for testing for hepatitis. All centrifugation should be carried out using sealed buckets or tubes. Disposable pipettes (e.g. one-piece plastic 'Movettes' (Nunc)) and/or autopipettes should be used at all stages, avoiding mouth pipetting.

4.3.3.2 *Serum.* Whole blood is collected into glass (specially treated to prevent haemolysis) or plastic tubes. The blood is allowed to clot by standing for several hours at room temperature or 4°C overnight. The clot is freed from the sides of the tube with a wooden or plastic applicator, and sedimented by centrifugation at 1500 *g* for 10 min. The serum is removed for storage frozen at $-40°C$ as aliquots in suitable tubes (as for rat tissue, there must not be too much air space, and the seal and labelling must be good at −40°C).

4.3.3.3 *Plasma*. Whole blood is placed in glass or plastic tubes containing anticoagulant (EDTA or lithium heparin) and mixed by inversion. The tubes are spun immediately at 1500 g for 10 min and the plasma is removed (avoiding buffy layer at interface) for storage frozen at −40°C. The stipulations for storage tubes are as for serum.

4.3.3.4 *Platelets*. Blood for platelets should contact only plastic or metal, not untreated glass. Twenty-millilitre samples of blood are collected in 30-ml plastic universal bottles containing 5 ml ACD (citric acid H_2O, 8 g; tri-sodium citrate $2H_2O$, 22 g; dextrose, 22.4 g/litre of water) as anti-coagulant. After centrifugation at 150 g for 15 min, the platelet-rich plasma is transferred using plastic pipettes to plastic centrifuge tubes and re-spun at 1500 g for 10 min. The sedimented platelets are then washed by being resuspended in 5 ml of isotonic saline; any red blood cells are removed by centrifugation at 150 g for 5 min. The platelets, after re-pelleting by centrifugation at 1500 g, are suspended in 1 ml of 0.2 M phosphate buffer at pH 7 for storage frozen. Membranes can be broken by freezing and thawing twice (e.g. for MAO or 5-HT analysis (Owen *et al.*, 1976; Joseph *et al.*, 1977)).

4.3.3.5 *Lymphocytes*. This procedure is a modification of that supplied with Ficoll-Paque by Pharmacia. Twenty millilitres of whole blood is collected into a sterile container without any anticoagulant and stirred gently with a wooden applicator for 15 min to remove the fibrin that adheres to the stick. The blood is now diluted with a half volume of medium RPMI 1640 containing HEPES buffer (Moore *et al.*, 1967) (at room temperature to avoid disruption of cells) and mixed gently by inversion. In a 15-ml plastic centrifuge tube (e.g. Falcon 209) an equal volume of blood is layered gently on to 'lymphocyte separation medium' (Ficoll Paque, Pharmacia Ltd). The tube is centrifuged at 2200 rpm for 25 min at room temperature (no brake). The upper serum layer is removed and the next layer, containing lymphocytes, is transferred to a clean tube containing a few millilitres of medium. The volume is made up to 20 ml and the contents are mixed by inversion. Centrifugation at 1500 rpm for 10 min and a further two washes are followed by final suspension in 0.5 ml of medium. Then, 0.5 ml of 10% DMSO is added dropwise with mixing.

The number of lymphoctyes retrieved and their viability are deter-mined by counting 10 μl of the suspension in 90 μl of 0.4% trypan blue using a haemocytometer counting chamber (Neubau). Viable cells are those that take up stain and/or contain viable internal structures. The final preparation should be diluted with a 1 : 1 mixture of medium : 10% DMSO to contain $1-1.5 \times 10^6$ lymphocytes per 0.2 ml. Aliquots are stored in suitable screw-topped containers in liquid nitrogen after first prefreezing at $-30°C$ for 30 min.

4.3.3.6 *White cells.* Heparinised blood is mixed in a syringe in the ratio of 4:1 (v/v) with 6% dextran (mol. wt. 100000–200000) in Earle's balanced salt solution. The syringe is suspended from a hook formed by bending the end of the needle, and the red cells are allowed to settle for 30 min at room temperature. The supernatant is carefully ejected through the needle into a tube and left for 5 min to check for any further sedimentation. The tube is centrifuged at 800 *g* for 10 min and the plasma/dextran is discarded. The cells are suspended in sterile water for 30 s (no longer) to destroy any remaining red cells. Osmolality is restored by adding and mixing an equal volume of 2.3% KCl. After spinning, the cells are washed twice with saline before final suspension and storage frozen.

4.4.4 *Human urine*
Collection of other than spot urines is most conveniently carried out in a single large container that will hold all the urine in the sample (for ease of mixing before sampling). Half-gallon (2½-litre) rectangular plastic bottles with screw caps (Raven RSC/2500) will take a 24-h urine sample except in unusual cases. Where subjects are supervising themselves, or a variety of personnel (e.g. nursing staff) are supervising, it is useful to have a detailed protocol for distribution (Fig. 4.2). Male subjects will be able to urinate directly into the bottles, but for female subjects, and for elderly, confused or psychologically disturbed, male subjects, collection should be made in a plastic jug for transfer to the container. The main container should be kept refrigerated during the collection, and mixed by inversion after each addition.

For some determinations, and especially where refrigeration is not possible, a preservative may be added to the bottle before the collection starts. Acid is commonly used to protect bases such as amines; 20 ml of 3 N HCl or 5 ml glacial acetic acid will bring the pH of a 24-h collection from its normal pH of about 5 to pH 1–2. However, care should be exercised in giving bottles containing neat acid (at the beginning of the collection) to psychiatric patients for obvious reasons. Other commonly used preservatives include 10 ml 10% EDTA, sodium metabisulphite as antioxidant or Bacitracin (0.45 mM final) (Sigma, Poole, England) to inhibit peptidases.

As soon as practicable after the last sample (conveniently in the

1 Collection is commenced by obtaining an 8.00 a.m. specimen which is discarded.

2 Subsequent collection should be made of all urine voided. When the patient wishes to empty his bowels it may be most convenient to ask him to urinate separately beforehand.

3 Urine should be immediately transferred to the collection bottle in the refrigerated cubicles on the ward, and the contents mixed by inversion. Do not fill the bottle to the brim; ask for another bottle or use any suitable bottle placed in the same cubicle.

4 Each 24-h period will terminate with an 8.00 a.m. specimen, which is placed in the same bottle.

Fig. 4.2.   24-hour Urine Collection Protocol

morning), the contents are thoroughly mixed, the volume is determined (can be by weight) and noted, and aliquots are taken for storage at −40°C. We use plastic Universals for storage of samples; the total urine volume and other details are recorded on the bottle as well as in a running log, and a code number from the log is written on the bottle label and cap.

References

Bird, E.D., Crow, T.J., Iversen, L.L., Longden, A., Mackay, A.V.P., Riley, G.J. and Spokes, E.G. (1979). Dopamine and homovanillic acid concentrations in post-mortem brain in schizophrenia. *J. Physiol.* **293**, 36−7P.

British Standards Institution (1975). British Standard 4851 (as amended), HMSO, London.

British Standards Institution (1979). British Standard 5726, HMSO, London.

Collins, C.H., Hartley, E.G. and Pilsworth, R. (1974). *The Prevention of Laboratory-acquired Infection.* PHLS Monograph Series No. 6 HMSO, London.

Cross, A.J. and Owen, F. (1979). The activities of glutamic acid decarboxylase and choline acetyltransferase in post mortem brains of schizophrenics and controls. *Biochem. Soc. Trans.* **7**, 145−6.

Crow, T.J., Owen, F., Cross, A.J., Johnstone, E.C., Joseph, M.H. and Longden, A. (1980). The dopamine receptor is the site of the primary disturbance in the type I syndrome of schizophrenia. In *Enzymes and Neurotransmitters in Mental Disease* (E. Usdin, T.L. Sourkes and M.B.H. Youdim, Eds), 559−72, Wiley, New York.

De Armond, S.J., Fusco, M.M. and Dewey, M.M. (1974). *Structure of the Human Brain; a Photographic Atlas*, Oxford University Press, New York.

Glowinski, J. and Iversen, L.L. (1966). Regional studies of catecholamines in the rat brain. I. The disposition of ^{3}H-norepinephrine, ^{3}H-dopamine and ^{3}H-dopa in various regions of the brain. *J. Neurochem.* **13**, 655−69.

Horn, A.S., Cuello, A.C. and Miller, R.J. (1974). Dopamine in the mesolimbic system of the rat brain: endogenous levels and the effects of drugs on the uptake mechanism and stimulation of adenylate cyclase activity. *J. Neurochem.* **22**, 265–70.

HMSO (1961). Human Tissues Act, HMSO, London.

Howie, J.M. (1978). Code of Practice for the Prevention of Infection in Clinical Laboratories and Post-mortem Rooms. Report of a Working Party Chaired by J.M. Howie. HMSO, London.

Joseph, M.H., Owen, F., Baker, H.F. and Bourne, R.C. (1977). Platelet serotonin concentration and monoamine oxidase activity in unmedicated chronic schizophrenic and in schizoaffective patients. *Psychol. Med.* **7**, 159–62.

Kiser, R.S. (1982). A simple method for obtaining chronic cerebrospinal fluid samples from awake rats. *Brain Res. Bull.* **8**, 787–9.

Moore, G.E., Gerner, R.E. and Franklin, H.A. (1967). Culture of normal human leucocytes. *J. Amer. Med. Assoc.* **199**, 519–24.

Owen, F., Bourne, R.C., Crow, T.J., Johnstone, E.C., Bailey, A.R. and Hershon, H.I. (1976). Platelet monoamine oxidase in schizophrenia: an investigation in drug-free chronic hospitalised patients. *Arch. Gen. Psychiat.* **33**, 1370–3.

Palkovits, M. (1973). Isolated removal of hypothalamic or other brain nuclei of the rat. *Brain Res.* **59**, 449–50.

Patten, J. (1977). *Neurological Differential Diagnosis*, Starke, London, 259–66.

Rodnight, R. (1975). Obtaining, fixing and extracting neural tissues. In *Practical Neurochemistry* (H. McIlwain, Ed.), 2nd edn, 1–16, Churchill Livingstone, Edinburgh.

Simpson, J.A. (1980). How to do a lumbar puncture. *Brit. J. Hosp. Med.* **24**, 384–5.

Tyrrell, D.A.J., Parry, R.P., Crow, T.J., Johnstone, E.C. and Ferrier, I.N. (1979). Possible virus in schizophrenia and some neurological disorders. *Lancet* **i**, 839–41.

Waddington, J.L. and Cross, A.J. (1978). Neurochemical changes following kainic acid lesions of the nucleus accumbens. *Life Sci.* **22**, 1011–14.

5 *Michael H. Joseph*

Analysis of the principal amine transmitters and their metabolites, with particular reference to HPLC methods

5.1 Introduction

An essential component in the study of the functional state of transmitters in the brain is the measurement of these neurotransmitters and their metabolites in tissues and physiological fluids. The principal monoamine transmitters in the brain (noradrenaline, dopamine and serotonin (5-hydroxytryptamine)) give rise to discrete metabolic products which do not re-enter general metabolism (in contrast to the amino acid transmitters, for example). Thus estimation of these amines and their metabolites in discrete areas of brain gives information on the amounts of the transmitters present, and also on their turnover. A typical question asked might be: to what extent has a lesion depleted one or more amines? Or, is a drug, an environmental manipulation or a disease state associated with altered metabolic activity of one or more amines, or with an altered pattern of metabolism?

In humans, the tissue of central interest to neuroscientists, psychiatrists and neurologists is rarely available except at post-mortem. In animal experiments also, financial or ethical considerations may limit the availability of brain tissue; for example, chronic rather than acute studies may be carried out. Amine metabolism can be studied via the cerebrospinal fluid (CSF); this requires an operation which is not simple in animals (see Chapter 4) and ethical considerations severely limit its availability in humans. Accordingly amines and their metabolites have been studied in blood and urine. This raises problems of interpretation, particularly the relative contributions of central and peripheral pools of amines. 3-Methoxy-4-hydroxyphenylglycol (MHPG or MOPEG) is the principal metabolite of noradrenaline in the brain but not in the periphery. Comparisons between the rate of production of MHPG by the brain and the rate of MHPG excretion in urine suggest that in primates, including man (Maas *et al.*, 1979), a very substantial proportion of MHPG excreted in urine derives from the brain (for review see DeMet and Halaris, 1979). More recent studies on peripheral metabolism of MHPG (Blomberry *et al.*, 1980; Mardh *et al.*, 1981, 1983) have thrown some doubt upon this interpretation, but MHPG is currently the blood and urinary metabolite most widely held to reflect brain metabolism of an amine, viz. noradrenaline.

The analytical problems derive from the low levels of the amines and metabolites either relatively in a complex mixture (brain amine content is one-thousandth of that of glutamate or ascorbate) or absolutely in a simpler mixture (parent amines in CSF). Analysis involves three stages, considered in this order below: extraction from tissue or fluid, separation, and detection and quantification. The second and third stages are mutually interdependent since more specific detection requires a lesser degree of separation and vice versa.

The metabolic relationships between the biogenic amines and their precursors are shown in Fig. 5.1, and those between the amines and their metabolites in Fig. 5.2. It can be seen that all three major amines are synthesised from aromatic amino acids by ring hydroxylation (A) (to DOPA and 5-HTP) and subsequent decarboxylation of the side chain (B). The metabolic products of the catecholamines are more numerous than those of 5-HT because of the occurrence of O-methylation in addition to the action of monoamine oxidase; these enzymes can act in either order (A+C or B).

All these species therefore, the biogenic amines and their metabolites and precursors, are aromatic molecules (hydrophobic) with aliphatic side chains with polar functional groups (hydrophilic). This partial hydrophobic nature is useful in selectively extracting and separating them, and their aromatic nature gives them physical properties useful in determining them, viz. fluorescence (of parent molecules or of simply prepared derivatives) and electrochemical activity.

Methods of determination based on tagging with labelled groups with relatively specific purified enzymes are not discussed in this chapter. Here the specificity is provided by the enzymic step, and the subsequent analytical problem is analogous to that for the determination of enzyme activity, that is, the separation of the labelled product from large amounts of (chemically dissimilar) labelled precursor, and also from small amounts of

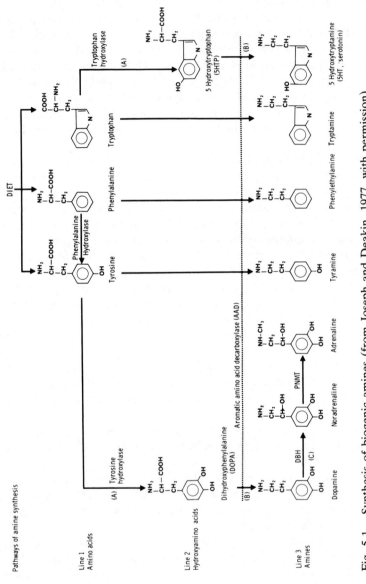

Fig. 5.1. Synthesis of biogenic amines (from Joseph and Deakin, 1977, with permission).

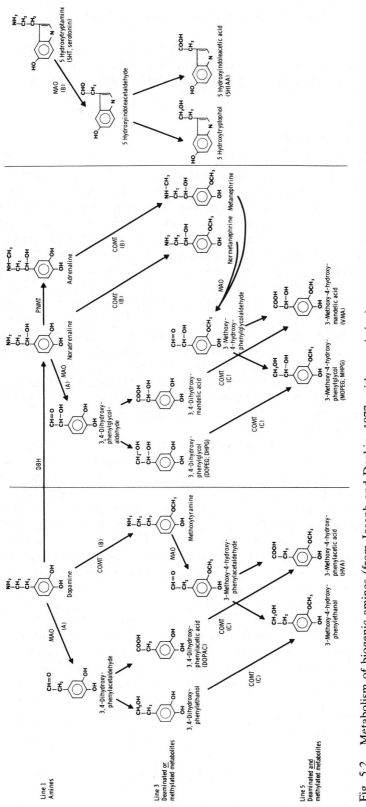

Fig. 5.2. Metabolism of biogenic amines (from Joseph and Deakin, 1977, with permission).

(chemically similar) other molecules labelled by the enzyme. The application of such methods to catecholamine determination is reviewed in relation to other techniques by Holly and Makin (1983) (see also section 5.4.1).

5.2 General procedures

5.2.1 *Extraction*

5.2.1.1 *Brain tissue.* As is general in the biochemical analysis of metabolites, the first stage involves efficient separation from protein and lipids into a fluid medium, while minimising enzymic or non-enzymic (e.g. oxidative) changes. In the case of tissue this involves disruption of fresh or frozen tissue into a protein precipitant in the cold (~4°C). Determination of the efficiency of the extraction is dealt with in section 5.2.2.

Since rapid precipitation of protein, and especially inactivation of enzymes, is required, homogenisation is usually in 5–10 volumes of a dilute solution of inorganic (0.1 N hydrochloric, 0.4 N perchloric (PCA)) or organic (10% ≃ 0.6 N trichloroacetic (TCA)) acids. We have also obtained adequate protein precipitation using citrate–phosphate buffer pH 3 (0.1 M citric acid +0.2 M sodium dihydrogen phosphate: Cross and Joseph, 1981). Amines and metabolites are also efficiently extracted into organic solvents; the use of acidified butanol (prepared by adding 0.85 ml conc. HCl per litre of *n*-butanol (Chang, 1964; Curzon and Green, 1970; Joseph and Baker, 1976) results in a particularly clear supernatant (see section 5.3.3 and Fig. 5.4).

Brain does not contain the structural elements present in muscle or liver, and thus is easily dispersed by hand homogenisation. For small amounts of brain tissue (~50 mg) we have used disposable plastic tubes (1.5 ml Sarstedt or equivalent) with a pestle made from a shaped glass rod. For larger amounts we use a mechanical homogeniser, with 10- or 30-ml thick-walled round-bottomed centrifuge tubes. It is important that the stainless steel shaft and blades of the homogeniser are compatible with the homogenisation medium for the particular assay. Acid media can dissolve metal ions which will interfere in fluorescence or electrochemical assays. Seals may not be compatible with certain organic solvents used. Any particular homogeniser will have to be tested in the actual method. We use an Ultra Turrax with shaft 2N (for small tubes) or 18N (large tubes), which have no seals in contact with the media and are compatible with the acid solvents mentioned previously. The Ultra Turrax shaft is cleaned thoroughly and run in medium alone and wiped before each sample is homogenised. Mechanical homogenisation generates aerosols and is therefore carried out in a fume cupboard, or in a B2-class containment facility for human or other primate brains where the risk of infection is greater (see Chapter 4).

The tubes containing the dispersant are pre-cooled to about 10°C, and the frozen sample is weighed in by difference on an electronic top-pan balance. After homogenisation, the tubes are stood in a 4°C refrigerator for 10 min to aid protein precipitation before removal of denatured protein by centrifugation at 2000–3000 g for 10–15 min in a standard small laboratory centrifuge (MSE Super Minor) or an Eppendorf centrifuge (5 min at 8000 g) for small samples.

If subsequent processing of the sample requires an acid solution, the supernatant can be used directly. If it is to be neutralised, then a reduction in the ionic strength may be desirable; this can be achieved for HCl extracts by freeze drying, for TCA extracts by ether extraction, which removes TCA, and for PCA extracts by neutralisation with a potassium salt, precipitating the insoluble $KClO_4$ (see Joseph and Halliday, 1975).

Standardisation by wet weight: the water content of the brain tissue will contribute a small but not negligible volume to the supernatant. The simplest way to allow for this, if the results are to be expressed per wet weight of tissue, is to make up the final dilutions of standard (mixture) such that a volume of water corresponding to that present in the tissue sample is added to the homogenisation medium with them (see section 5.2.2). A sufficient approximation to this for brain tissue is 80% (w/w).

Alternatively this can be allowed for in brain by taking x ml of supernatant as deriving from $x/(V + 0.8 \text{ g})$ of the weight of tissue taken, where: V = volume of homogenisation medium (ml), and g = weight of tissue taken (grams). This consideration underlines the importance of storage of brain samples in such a way that they cannot gain or lose water (Chapter 4). (If dehydration or condensation has occurred, the results must be expressed relative to a tissue marker, e.g. protein or DNA content measured in the same sample.)

5.2.1.2 *Blood*

(a) *Plasma and serum.* Being a fluid, extraction of plasma or serum can be achieved simply by thorough mixing with a protein precipitant in a centrifuge tube (e.g. 15 ml conical or 1.5 ml plastic disposable). The high viscosity of blood fractions requires careful control of sampler operation and vigorous mixing on a vortex mixer. Since quantification is normally with reference to volume (water content assumed 100%), aliquots of plasma or serum can be dispensed before freezing for storage. This helps to prevent chemical changes associated with repeated thawing and freezing. If aliquots are to be taken after unfreezing, removal of precipitated fibrin by a short centrifugation is convenient.

Common protein precipitants for blood plasma or serum include those mentioned for brain. Other organic acids have been specified for particular purposes; picric acid (1% w/v) or sulphosalicylic acid (3% w/v) (Rodnight, 1975). Duggan and Udenfriend (1956) specify tungstic acid, generated *in situ* by adding 2 ml of water to 0.5 ml of plasma, followed by 0.25 ml of 0.6N sulphuric acid, and 0.25 ml 10% (w/v) sodium tungstate successively with mixing. Acid butanol is effective for plasma at 5–10 volumes (Joseph and Baker, 1976) as is 4 volumes of methanol (Joseph and Davies, 1983). Precipitated protein is removed by centrifugation after standing in the cold as previously described. Blanchard (1981) has usefully reviewed the extent of protein removal by adding varying proportions of these agents. Lipid rejection and recovery of metabolites are clearly also important.

(b) *Whole blood.* The main problems with determinations in whole blood are its viscosity, and poor recoveries of 5-HT, particularly because of the tendency of haemoglobin to oxidise 5-HT during the precipitation of protein. The latter problems are overcome in the method of Geeraerts *et al.* (1974) by dispensing a measured volume of whole blood into an antioxidant solution before freezing. In our modification (Joseph, 1978a), 1 ml of heparinised whole blood is taken up into a fresh disposable 1 ml syringe, squirted into 0.1 ml of a solution of 3 g ascorbic acid and 15 g EDTA per 100 ml water in an Eppendorf disposable 1.5 ml tube and snap-frozen in liquid nitrogen. For analysis the sample is thawed and diluted with 2.5 ml of water to complete haemolysis. Efficient recovery of 5-HT is obtained by protein precipitation with alkaline zinc sulphate. One millilitre of 10% $ZnSO_4$ and 0.5 ml 1.0N NaOH are added successively with mixing.

(c) *Platelets.* Separation of platelets is described in Chapter 4. Platelet suspensions can be extracted with acid butanol after freezing and thawing at least twice (Joseph *et al.*, 1977).

5.2.1.3 *Cerebrospinal fluid and urine.* As aqueous solutions, normally with low protein content, these are easier to deal with from the point of view of extraction. CSF is used directly in most assays, the major analytical problem being the low levels of metabolites, especially the parent amines. Removal of cellular matter and proteins, together with any potentially infectious agents without dilution, is conveniently achieved by filtration using a bench centrifuge. We have had tube supports made up for this purpose from Delrin (a nylon plastic) and perspex rods, which enable disposable Eppendorf tubes to be used for the sample and filtrate facilitating prior and subsequent storage (Fig. 5.3). Similar devices, either disposable or not, are commercially available (Micropartition system and Centrifee, Amicon, Woking, UK, or Centrifugal Microfilter; Anachem, Luton, UK for Bioanalytical Systems. West Lafayette, Indiana, USA).

In the case of urine, the amine metabolites are more abundant, and

Centrifugal ultrafilter

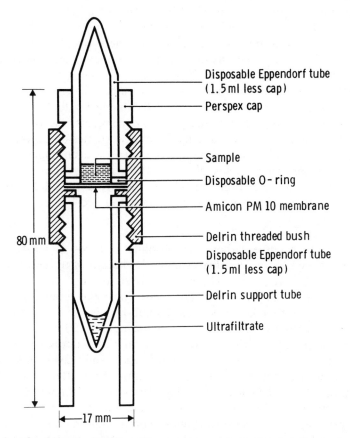

Fig. 5.3.   Centrifugal ultrafilter. The perspex cap is inverted over a rack, and an Eppendorf tube with the cap trimmed off is placed in it. The sample is placed in this tube which is then covered with the O-ring from a Nunc disposable 2 ml screw-cap tube. A 12 mm disc cut from a sheet of Amicon PM10 membrane is secured shiny side down by screwing on the threaded bush. A second Eppendorf tube minus cap is placed in the support tube and screwed on. The whole is spun in a standard 15 ml centrifuge bucket for about 20 min at about 2000 *g*. (From Joseph *et al.*, 1981c, with permission).

thus the major analytical problems are high concentrations of salts and of other metabolic products. Interfering drug metabolites can be a particular problem when dealing with human samples. Neutral amine metabolites can readily be extracted into organic solvents (see section 5.4.2.3), and at acid pH acidic metabolites are also extracted (section 5.4.3.3(b).

Catecholamines are normally extracted on to alumina (section 5.4.3.4) and 5-HT is extracted at alkaline pH (section 5.3.2).

Collection and preservation of 24-h samples of urine is described in Chapter 4. Results from urine analysis are not normally presented as concentrations but as amounts per 24 h or per hour over a specified time period. To allow for variations in body mass, urinary excretion is some-times expressed as a ratio to that of creatinine. However, this compounds the variability of the metabolite of interest with the inter-subject variability of creatinine excretion. It is a useful technique for looking at intra-subject variation (repeated samples) if the completeness of the 24-h samples is in question. This is usually the case in studies on psychiatric or confused patients and it may be necessary to express even single results in this way (see, for example, Joseph *et al.*, 1976, 1979). Alternatively total apparent creatinine excretion can be used as an additional criterion to exclude certain samples from analysis (Fawcett *et al.*, 1972).

5.2.2 *Use of standard solutions*

Because of the relative rather than absolute methods of measurement used in the assays to be described, standard solutions of the substances to be measured are required. These are carried through the method in parallel with the samples to be analysed. Since the amines and their metabolites are rather labile, standard solutions are best kept frozen at temperatures similar to those of the stored samples (-20 to $-70°C$). The frozen stock standard (which may have multiple components) is more stable, particularly in respect of repeated freezing and thawing if stored at 100 times the strength required: fresh dilutions of 50-, 100- and 200-fold can then be prepared each working day. The stability of amine standards may be enhanced if they are made up in dilute acid.

As previously noted, these working standard dilutions can be made up in a volume corresponding to the volume of tissue water in the sample. Thus 100 mg of brain containing 250 ng/g 5-HT, say, will be represented by 25 ng 5-HT in $100 \times 0.8 = 80$ μl of water. This is particularly important where organic solvents are used for extraction, since a part of the tissue water is extracted. With acid butanol, for instance (see sections 5.3.2 and 5.3.3), a part of this tissue water is displaced back into the dilute acid phase at the first extraction step. Since the latter volume is usually not very much greater than the former, the potential error is quite serious.

It is then good practice to take the three standards mentioned above, together with a suitable blank, through the method with each batch of samples. This provides a routine check on linearity of response. The sum of the respective differences of the three standards from the blank divided by 3.5 ($= 0.5 + 1 + 2$) will then give a weighted average of the response factor for the middle standard which will be used to calculate the results if a linear calibration is achieved. As this implies, in setting up a method, standard solutions will be used to determine the relationship between concentration and response of the measuring instrument over a range wider than that likely to be encountered in the samples. A linear calibration is normally sought.

The extraction and each of the separation steps in the method will have a proportional recovery associated with it, and this should be independent of concentration. Thus out of ten units initially present in the brain sample, eight may get into the extract and seven of these into the final solution to be derivatised and quantified, after allowing for known physical losses (due, for example, to taking a known volume less than that into which the sample was extracted). In this example the recovery of the extraction will be 80%, of the separation $700/8 = 87.5\%$, and the overall recovery 70%. Unfortunately the term 'recovery' is used to describe both the first and the second figure.

Recovery of the extraction can be determined by dividing a homogenate and a blank in two and adding standard to one of each pair and an equal volume of water to the other of each pair. The recovery of the extraction is then given by

$$\frac{(\text{sample} + \text{standard}) - (\text{sample} + \text{water})}{(\text{blank} + \text{standerd}) - (\text{blank} + \text{water})} \times 100\%$$

This illustrates the problem with naturally occurring metabolites, as opposed to drugs, that recovery at the level actually found in the tissue cannot be determined. Recovery can only be determined after significantly elevating the endogenous content. Sometimes tissue from other regions containing low levels, e.g. cerebellum, can be used, but then recovery is not measured from the same environment.

Recovery of the separation can be determined by comparison of a standard solution taken through the method with one used directly for the final stage. If there are problems with overall recovery of the separation, the recovery can be determined successively at each step *preceding* the latest one at which the pure substance can be determined by direct addition (i.e. going back stepwise through the method).

Low recoveries at the extraction or separation stages may still yield a usable method if they are consistent and independent of concentration. Even inconsistent recoveries across samples can be dealt with by using internal standardisation for each unknown (spiking), but this will entail double the amount of analytical work. Low apparent recoveries may also be due to interfering substances from reagents or from tissue coming through the method; addition of standards to one half and water to the other half of the final stage of a processed sample or blank will enable this possibility to be assessed.

Once linearity and recovery are established, the method can be checked for independence from the effect of tissue concentration (the apparent concentration should reduce in direct proportion to the dilution of the homogenate). Validity is then examined by comparison with results in the literature. One caveat here is that results in the literature may or may not be corrected for recovery. Needless to say in the ideal world all papers presenting analytical results would state whether or not the results given were corrected for recovery, and which sort of recovery was meant.

5.2.3 *Precautions during work-up procedures*

As noted in the previous sections, in the analysis of amines and metabolites we are dealing with minute amounts (concentrations in the range of 1 ppm to 10 ppb) of relatively unstable compounds. It is desirable that samples should be stored as intact tissue, etc. If samples are homogenised and stored for subsequent analysis, a minimal requirement is that standard solutions are stored under the same conditions (same temperature, same medium). Even better practice is to include recovery samples (homogenates stored with and without known amounts of added standards) as well as standard solutions.

It is advisable to avoid excessive exposure to ultraviolet light (especially direct sunlight) and prolonged exposure to room temperatures or above (e.g. in a centrifuge warmed by use). Delays during the separation should be kept to a minimum especially when samples are at extremes of pH or elevated temperatures. Where delays do occur, samples should be kept in the 4°C refrigerator. However, this must be balanced against delays due to the time to re-equilibrate to room temperature so that volumetric errors are not made as samples sequentially warm up.

Samples required to be kept overnight during a separation should be placed in a −20 to −40°C freezer, in an aqueous medium if possible and avoiding extremes of pH. Running standards and blanks in parallel with samples helps to allow for changes but these may be more (or less) marked in the samples than in the standards.

The final products of the *o*-phthalaldehyde (OPT) reaction for 5-hydroxyindoles (section 5.3) and of the TFAA reaction for MHPG (section 5.4.2.2) can be kept in the refrigerator overnight, but the effect of freezing is unknown. Samples for injection into the HPLC are normally in mild aqueous solutions, and can be frozen until required (but repeated freezing and thawing should be avoided here and in general).

5.3 Analysis of serotonin (5-HT) and related 5-hydroxyindoles by fluorescence

5.3.1 *Introduction: fluorescence analysis*

In analytical biochemistry, many substances can be determined by light absorption using spectrophotometry, the logarithm of the intensity of transmitted light at a particular wavelength being inversely proportional to concentration. In biological materials the relative abundance of amines and their metabolites is too low for direct spectrophotometry to be useful, although methods based on the formation of more strongly absorbing derivatives (Udenfriend *et al.*, 1955) are used in clinical chemistry laboratories for estimation of 5-HIAA in urine. An extremely useful physical property shared by all indoles is that of fluorescence; indeed their fluorescence was a major factor in the development of fluorescence analysis in biochemistry. Fluorescence analysis is in general more specific than spectrophotometry because the wavelength of the incident light, as well as the (longer) wavelength of the light emitted (normally measured at right angles), is specified. This difference in wavelength means that scattered light does not interfere, resulting in higher signal-to-noise ratios and thus higher sensitivities. A good general text on fluorescence analysis is provided by Udenfriend (1962, 1969).

The high degree of specificity conferred by the small number of compounds absorbing and emitting at the maxima for the indoles means in practice that the only separation required for measurement of any one indole is from other indoles. At the optimum wavelengths for indoles (excitation 280 nm/emission 330 nm) virtually all the fluorescence in many biological materials (in particular deproteinised plasma) is from unconjugated tryptophan, the indole-containing amino acid, itself the precursor of the 5-hydroxylated indoles. Thus tryptophan can be determined in plasma simply from the fluorescence of a deproteinised supernatant (Duggan and Udenfriend, 1956).

Udenfriend's group reported that 5-hydroxylated indoles showed a shift of emission wavelength to 550 nm in strongly acid solution (for instance 3N HCl). 5-Hydroxytryptophan, the immediate precursor of 5-HT, is normally present in vanishingly small concentration in biological materials, except after direct administration of 5-HTP or after drug treatments (e.g. with aromatic amino acid decarboxylase inhibitors such as carbidopa). Thus in particular tissues where either 5-HT (platelets) or 5-HIAA (CSF) are in great preponderance, fluorescence determination can be done at 280/550 nm on an acidified deproteinised extract (Korf and Valkenburgh-Sikkema, 1969; Geeraerts *et al.*, 1974; Joseph, 1978a; and see section 5.5.2). In other tissues, such as brain, where both are present, then 5-HT and 5-HIAA must first be separated. Where concentrations are low, or determinations on small samples are sought, the 5-hydroxyindole fluorescence can be amplified. Ninhydrin will react with 5-HT but not with non-amine 5-hydroxyindoles to give a more fluorescent product (Vanable, 1963; Snyder *et al.*, 1965). An alternative derivatisation is common to all 5-hydroxyindoles, but not to unsubstituted indoles (Maickel and Miller, 1966). *o*-Phthalaldehyde (OPT) reacts with primary amines (including amino acids) at alkaline pH and room temperature. The specific 5-hydroxyindole reaction, however, is carried out in strongly acid solution yielding a product with strong fluorescence maxima at 360/ 470 nm. This is the derivatisation used in the methods to be described here.

Note on instrumentation for fluorescence analysis. An analytical spectrofluorimeter is required. We have used the Perkin Elmer MPF-3a, with diffraction grating monochromators for control of excitation and emission wavelengths. Either can be driven in synchrony with the chart so that spectra rather than peak height only are routinely obtained. The instrument is equipped with a wide-spectrum xenon arc lamp and has a ratio mode to allow for lamp instability. It would, however, be improved by ratioing the final emitted light to that emerging from, rather than that entering, the excitation monochromator, permitting absolute spectra which are reproducible from machine to machine to be recorded. These specifications can be contrasted with those given for an HPLC detection instrument in section 5.4.3.2(d).

5.3.2 *Separation*

If native or derived 5-hydroxyindole fluorescence is used, then the separation problem usually reduces to the separation of 5-HT and 5-HIAA. Tissues containing both, e.g. brain, contain insignificant concentrations of the other two 5-hydroxyindoles, 5-HTP and 5-hydroxytryptophol, except after 5-HTP or drug administration. Solvent extraction is a convenient method of separating biogenic amines and metabolites, amines being extractable into an organic phase at alkaline pH, at which they are uncharged, and acids conversely being extractable at acid pH at which they are uncharged. The same general considerations apply to catecholamines and metabolites, with the proviso that the catechol group is rather readily oxidised at pH values above 8. Thus 5-HT and 5-HIAA can be sequentially extracted at alkaline and acid pH as in the procedure of Udenfriend *et al.* (1958), leaving 5-HTP, if present, in the residual aqueous phase. In the procedure to be described for brain, the use of acid butanol as extractant and protein precipitant provides a particularly clean organic supernatant from which amines (here 5-HT) and acids (here 5-HIAA) are sequentially back-extracted at acid and neutral pH respectively. Amino acids will also be extracted into the acid phase, in which tryptophan and kynurenine can be readily determined by specific reactions (Joseph, 1978a,b). If present, 5-HTP will interfere with the 5-HT determination, but 5-HT can be extracted, after neutralising the acid, with an organic soluble ion-pairing agent such as diethylhexylphosphoric acid (DEHPA) or Kalignost (tetra-phenyl boron) and subsequently recovered in dilute acid again, leaving 5-HTP in the aqueous phase (Joseph and Baker, 1976).

5.3.3 *Procedure*

This is shown in Fig. 5.4, and is modified from the procedure of Curzon and Green (1970) as described in Joseph and Baker (1976) and Joseph (1978a). If brain samples are stored at −40°C, then a series of brain samples can be weighed (by difference) into a series of tubes containing 5 volumes of acid butanol, which will be cooled by the samples. As the samples warm to 0–5°C they can be homogenised. We use an Ultra Turrax fitted with a shaft resistant to organic solvents and acids, cleaning it by running in acid butanol medium between samples. After 10 min at 4°C, precipitated protein is sedimented in a bench centrifuge (~2500 g), and a convenient volume of the supernatant (say 4.5 volumes) is removed to a stoppered tube for back-extraction with acid. Heptane is added to the organic phase to render it less polar. We have omitted cysteine from the acid phase because we found interference with subsequent tryptophan assay, but add it at the stage of 5-hydroxyindole derivative formation. After hand or mechanical shaking for a few minutes and brief centrifugation to aid separation of the phases, the volume of the lower (aqueous) phase is found to have been increased by the volume of brain water taken into the acid butanol and displaced by the heptane. In addition a disc of tissue debris is found at the interface. We then remove an appropriate volume of the organic phase to a second stoppered tube for the neutral extraction, displace the tissue disc to one side, and remove a fixed volume (say 1.2 ml) of the aqueous phase with a single pipette or sampler. This is placed in a fresh tube for subdivision, aliquots being taken for tryptophan and 5-HT estimation, and the residue processed for kynurenine if desired. If 5-HTP is present, it will also appear in this phase. 5-HT can then be separated by extraction into an organic phase with the aid of DEHPA, a cation exchange agent which is soluble in the organic phase. The acid solution is first neutralised (pH 7.0) and then extracted with 0.1M DE-HPA in chloroform. 5-HTP remains in the (upper) aqueous layer, in which it can be determined by the OPT reaction for 5-hydroxyindoles as described below. 5-HT is then recovered from the chloroform phase by acid extraction. Where volumes are sufficiently small, these extractions can be carried out in Eppendorf tubes. Where greater than 1 ml total volume but less than 5 ml, a 10 ml conical centrifuge tube held on to a vortex mixer *gripped at least* 2 cm *below the top* is convenient and saves on stoppered tubes.

Suitable aliquots (often 0.3 ml) of the acid phase containing 5-HT or the neutral phase containing 5-HTP are derivatised by placing in an Eppendorf tube and adding 0.65 ml of a freshly prepared solution of OPT

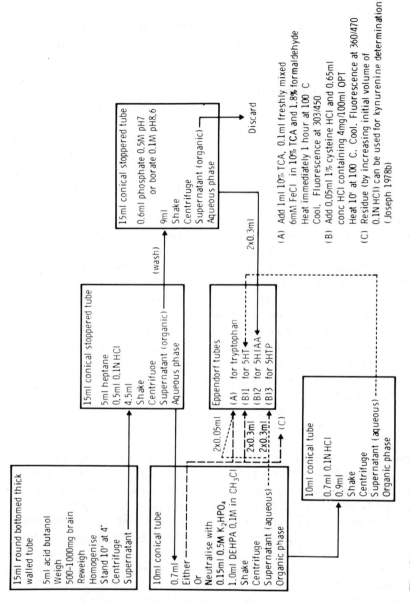

Fig. 5.4. Analytical scheme for fluorescence analysis of 5-HT and related indoles.

(4 mg/100 ml conc. HCl) and 0.05 ml of freshly prepared 1% cysteine hydrochloride solution. These are most conveniently prepared by making up OPT at 4 mg/1 ml conc. HCl and diluting 100-fold in conc. HCl to give sufficient for the number of samples, adding one-thirteenth of the volume of a 10 mg/ml solution of cysteine hydrochloride in water, mixing and adding 0.7 ml to each tube. After addition of reagents and mixing, the cap of each tube is pierced with a fine needle and the tubes are heated in a heating block with appropriate drillings. After cooling, the fluorescent. products may be kept in the +4°C refrigerator overnight before reading fluorescence at room temperature.

The neutral extract from the butanol–heptane is processed in exactly the same way for 5-HIAA determination. Removal of the organic phase following the neutral extraction is most simply achieved with a water-pump vacuum line and a pasteur pipette. Duplicate aliquots of the aqueous phase are then treated for 5-HIAA estimation. The procedure of Curzon and Green (1970) uses one of the aliquots as a tissue blank by destroying 5-HIAA with periodate before derivatising, as in the method of Korf and Valkenburgh–Sikkema (1969) from which they adapted it. However, this was necessary only because the latter authors were using urine and CSF; our experience has been that brain samples contribute no appreciable blank and that the sample is better utilised to provide duplicate determinations.

If follows from the rationale of the procedure that incomplete, or incomplete specificity of, extraction can result in cross-contamination of the fractions. In applying this method to the estimation of 5-HTP, 5-HT and 5-HIAA in plasma following 5-HTP administration, we found this to be of the order of 5% (Joseph and Baker, 1976, Table 1) after washing the butanol–heptane phase with 0.1N HCl before doing the neutral extraction. ·

5.3.4 *Trouble shooting*
Fluorescence procedures are fairly straightforward once it is appreciated that extremely small amounts of material are being measured and that fluorescence is readily quenched by minute traces of contaminants. Since the OPT condensation is performed in strong hydrochloric acid, contamination with metal ions or plasticiser from plastic laboratory ware are obvious hazards. As previously noted, trouble shooting should start at the last step and work backwards.

The first source of contamination is the water or reagents used. Often single distilled water is sufficiently pure, but in some laboratories double distillation or reverse osmosis purification is regarded as mandatory. Storage of the purified water may also lead to problems especially where plastic carboys or washbottles from which plasticiser may leach, are used.

In evaluating water contamination, access to alternative sources of purified water is helpful, as can be the availability of 'AnalaR' or 'HPLC' water from commercial suppliers. Normal biochemically clean glassware (detergent wash, copious cold rinsing, copious distilled water rinsing) is often adequate, but an acid wash before distilled water rinsing is used in many laboratories. Plastic ware should be regarded with suspicion until proved in the method. For the final stage of heating to form the OPT derivative in concentrated HCl, we have found that many 1.5 ml plastic disposable tubes yield a marked yellow colour in the solution, and we invariably use Eppendorf tubes for this step. Plasticiser from sampler tips can also be a problem.

Turning to reagents, we have encountered problems with some commercial samples of OPT. Sigma OPT has usually been satisfactory in our hands as have Sigma standards of 5-hydroxyindoles. Cysteine HCl (BDH) has not been a problem except as mentioned in tryptophan determination.

So far we have covered problems which may arise even in taking standard 5-hydroxyindole solutions through the last stage to produce a fluorescent product. If then there are problems with carrying standards through the entire method, these can arise from contaminants, initially in reagents, which go on through the method and interfere directly or degrade the compounds being measured. The organic reagents used (butanol, heptane) are prime candidates because relatively large volumes are extracted with small volumes of aqueous solutions. Here we have found it more efficient to shop around among suppliers than to redistil or wash problematic solvents.

The homogeniser used may be critical. The metal parts/plastic seals come into contact with the acid/organic extractants. We have had success with the Ultra Turrax with the 2N and 18N stainless steel shafts which have no seals, but a commercial blender resulted in unacceptable metal contamination.

5.4 Catecholamines and metabolites

5.4.1 *Introduction*

The native fluorescence of the catecholamines and their metabolites is much less than that of the indoles. For this reason fluorescence procedures for dopamine and for noradrenaline and adrenaline have used oxidation to the fluorescent dihydroxy indole and trihydroxyindole compounds respectively (Udenfriend, 1962; Atack, 1977). Fluorescence procedures for the principal dopamine metabolites HVA and DOPAC utilise alkaline ferricyanide oxidation to a fluorescent dimer and ethylene diamine condensation (a reaction common to all catechols), respectively

(Murphy *et al.*, 1969; Udenfriend, 1969). The principal metabolites of noradrenaline found in the brain are the neutral glycols MHPG and DHPG. As described in section 5.1.1, MHPG has attracted special interest as a monoamine metabolite found in plasma and urine which (in primates at least) may derive substantially from brain noradrenaline metabolism, peripheral noradrenaline being metabolished primarily to VMA. Meek and Neff (1972) described a fluorescence procedure for MHPG. However, this is not suitable for urine, and the ethylene diamine used for condensation needs frequent re-purification. Accordingly GLC or GC–MS are widely used as techniques for determination of MHPG, especially in plasma or urine. The agreement between these two methods is quite good (Muscettola *et al.*, 1981).

As noted previously, catechols are readily oxidised above pH 8 and thus solvent extraction at alkaline pH is not used for separation in the way described for 5-HT. Absorption on to alumina at neutral pH, in small columns or batch-wise, with subsequent acid elution is the most commonly used method of separation for catecholamines (Kissinger *et al.*, 1981; Mefford, 1981). Acid or neutral metabolites which retain the catechol grouping (DOPAC, DHPG) will also be extracted by alumina, but *o*-methylated ones (HVA, MHPG, normetadrenaline) will not. Determination of the catechols following elution may be by HPLC (see section 5.4.3.4) or by radioenzymic assay (Coyle and Henry, 1973; Saller and Zigmond, 1978; Baker and Johnson, 1981).

Alternatively, acid metabolites (DOPAC, HVA, VMA) are organic-extractable at acid pH. Neutral metabolites (MHPG, DHPG) are also extractable over a wide pH range in their free form. However, both glycols are found extensively sulphoconjugated in rat brain and CSF. In primate brain and CSF the free form predominates, but in urine from all species the conjugated forms (sulphate and glucuronide) predominate. This results in problems of separation since the hydrophilic conjugate is not readily extracted, and column separation techniques give rather unpredictable retention times. Most workers have therefore hydrolysed conjugates of MHPG and then determined the free form following extraction. Deconjugation will therefore be described in the next section.

5.4.2 *GLC analysis of MHPG*
5.4.2.1 *Deconjugation.* Acid hydrolysis of conjugates is the standard method for most compounds, but DHPG and MHPG are reported to be unstable under these conditions. Enzymic deconjugation is the alternative usually adopted. Crude enzyme preparations from the snail *Helix pomatia* (glusulase, helicase) are sometimes associated with the introduction of interfering compounds and/or substantial amounts of MHPG itself. If one is interested in the relative proportions of each of the sulphatase and

glucuronide conjugates, then more purified preparations containing either glucuronidase or sulphatase activity are required. We have confirmed that bacterial glucuronidase (ex *Escherischia Coli*, Sigma) shows no activity towards pure MHPG sulphate (courtesy of Roche Products), but we have not always found the converse for aryl sulphatase (Boehringer) purified from helicase. Accordingly we analyse three parallel samples, one unincubated (A), one with glucuronidase alone (B) and one with a mixture of glucuronidase and sulphatase (C). This gives free MHPG (A); sulphate (C–B) and glucuronide (B–A) are obtained by difference. Recently it has been suggested that dilute acid hydrolysis of MHPG-sulphate in brain under mild conditions may not in fact degrade MHPG; this would then get round problems of uncertainty of the extent of enzyme action, batch-to-batch variation and possible poisoning of enzymes by drugs or their metabolites found in the samples; the application of this technique to urine is currently under investigation.

5.4.2.2 *Rationale.* GLC separations are based on the partition of a volatile substance between a gas phase and a liquid phase coated on to a solid support. Thus a characteristic retention time is observed when this substance is volatilised into a stream of gas flowing down a packed column at a defined temperature. For a given column, retention time is governed primarily by volatility, and thus retention times will generally be shortened by raising the column temperature. For a polar substance such as MHPG a volatile derivative is prepared as follows.

After hydrolysis free MHPG is extracted into ethyl acetate at the pH of the hydrolysis buffer (extraction being substantially pH independent). Acetylation with acetic anhydride under alkaline aqueous conditions results in acetylation of the ring 4-hydroxyl, but not of the side-chain hydroxyls. Acetyl-MHPG is then extractable into the more hydrophobic dichloromethane, resulting in separation from relatively more hydrophilic interfering substances. Trifluoroacetylation of the side-chain hydroxyls using trifluoroacetic anhydride (TFAA) in organic solution yields a volatile derivative suitable for GLC with electron-capture detection (due to the halogen atoms). This derivative is also more stable than the tri-trifluoroacetyl derivative used by other workers (e.g. Dekirmenjian and Maas, 1970).

5.4.2.3 *Procedure.* Our procedure is quite fully described by Joseph *et al.* (1976) and by Walter and Shilcock (1977) and is therefore only summarised here. Hydrolysis with the enzyme combinations already described is carried out overnight in a 37°C heating block using glass-stoppered centrifuge tubes for simplicity of extraction the following day. Urine samples without enzymes but with added standard are carried through the method as recoveries of MHPG added to urine are higher than those added to water. However, recovery is consistent between urines, and hence a few samples with and without added standard can be used as standards for a batch of determinations. The unhydrolysed samples and samples plus standards are kept at 4°C overnight; buffer as for the enzymes is added and they are extracted in parallel with the incubates with two successive aliquots of ethyl acetate. The organic solvent is then removed from the pooled supernatants using a stream of dry, oxygen-free nitrogen. The conical tubes containing the supernatants are placed in a heating block at 37°C to assist evaporation, and the nitrogen is played on to the surface of the ethyl acetate via pasteur pipettes attached to a glass manifold with the same layout as the heating block. Alkaline aqueous acetylation of the MHPG is followed by extraction with dichloromethane (note: heavier than water). The dichloromethane is dried with anhydrous sodium sulphate, and the solvent is removed under nitrogen stream. Dryness is essential for the final step of trifluoracetylation in ethyl acetate, as is subsequent removal of all traces of excess TFAA under a nitrogen stream which will otherwise give a large unretained peak on chromotography. In addition to the Perkin-Elmer F30 with 6 ft SE301 column (Joseph *et al.*, 1976) we have also used a Hewlett-Packard 5713 with argon–methane carrier gas and 3 ft OV1 column and a Pye Unicam GCD with 1.5 m OV1 column. Figure 5.5 shows traces obtained with the last-mentioned instrument for total MHPG in two urine samples with and without added MHPG standard.

5.4.2.4 *Trouble shooting.* The sensitivity of electron capture detection renders it much more susceptible to carrier gas contamination and column bleed. One reason for using argon–methane in place of nitrogen in spite of its greater expense and lower sensitivity is that quality control is sometimes better, because it is made up as a special gas mixture. Gas purification pellets may require frequent changing, and columns may require prolonged conditioning before use, and reconditioning if any packing is subsequently added. Since the MHPG derivative is relatively unstable, glass columns are mandatory. Chromatograph design using metal capillary tubing, especially leading to the column, should be avoided. Active sites on the glass wall of the column can be inactivated by periodic injection of a commercially available silating agent. We have also found it useful to operate the detector at a rather high temperature (300°C) which discourages deposition of material, thus avoiding contamination and the need for frequent cleaning.

The first step is to obtain a sharp and reproducible response from injection of the internal standard in ethyl acetate. Solvent purity may be a problem. Again we have found it more economical to shop around for

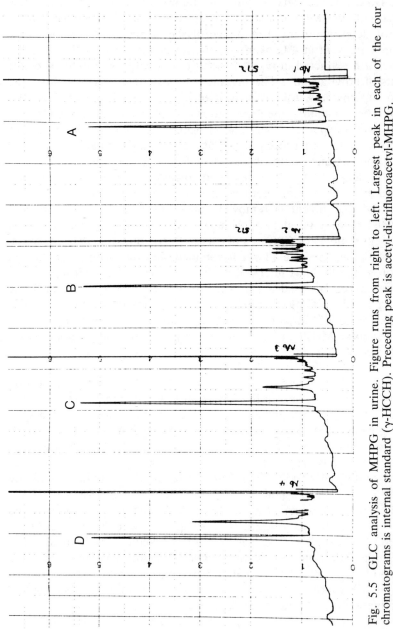

Fig. 5.5 GLC analysis of MHPG in urine. Figure runs from right to left. Largest peak in each of the four chromatograms is internal standard (γ-HCCH). Preceding peak is acetyl-di-trifluoroacetyl-MHPG. A and C are from two hydrolysed urine samples; B and D are the same urines respectively spiked with authentic MHPG.

reagents than to repurify them. Ethyl acetate from Reeve Angel (CT grade) and BDH (chromatography grade) have proved satisfactory.

The next step is to obtain a peak from pure MHPG standard. Since most of the procedure is the preparation of the determinable derivative, it is difficult to adopt a stepwise approach to disentangle problems encountered subsequent to the ethyl acetate extraction. (This emphasises the attraction of the HPLC methods in which the parent compound is determined as described in the next section.) The presence of interfering peaks in the TFAA can be detected by adding it to ethyl acetate, drying down, taking up in ethyl acetate and injecting. Another useful check on the TFAA is to make a simply prepared derivative to check whether a peak is obtained. *o*-Aminoacetophenone, the product of the method for kynurenine (Joseph, 1978b) is commercially available (Koch-Light) and a butyl acetate solution of it can be reacted with TFAA directly, excess reagent being hydrolysed and removed by extracting with an alkaline borate buffer. The organic supernatant can then be separated and directly injected.

Problems arising in the preparation of the MHPG derivative can then come from the other reagents used (methylene chloride, acetic anhydride) or inadequate removal of water before drying down for trifluoracetylation.

5.4.3 *HPLC Analysis of catecholamines and metabolites*
5.4.3.1 *Introduction.* The need to prepare derivatives of catecholamines and metabolites for fluorescence or GLC analysis, with correspondingly elaborate work-ups yielding results for only one or two compounds at once, emphasises the attraction of methods in which these compounds are separated and determined in their native form. Reversed-phase HPLC has recently enjoyed a surge of interest because of its ability to separate a wide range of different chemical species, with good separation of closely related compounds due to the high resolution of modern microparticulate packings. In liquid chromatography, a compound is characterised by the time it takes to migrate through a permeable solid (stationary) phase subjected to a flow of a liquid (mobile) phase. The term 'reversed phase' refers to a reversal of the normal situation in paper, thin layer or column chromatography in which the retention of a compound is determined by partition between a polar stationary phase and a non-polar mobile phase. In reversed-phase HPLC the microparticulate silica column packing has been rendered hydrophobic by reacting exposed silanol groups with alkyl silanes of some particular chain length. In use partition occurs between the hydrophobic (non-polar) alkyl chains on the stationary phase and the relatively hydrophilic (polar) eluting agent (usually an aqueous buffer). From the structures of the biogenic amines and metabolites (Figs. 5.1 and 5.2) it can be seen that the aromatic portions are modified by hydrophilic

substituents and side chains; this leads to good chromatography on reversed phase. The order of elution is the converse of that in normal phase chromatography, i.e. the most polar species elute first and the least polar last. Good control of retention time for a given column can then be achieved by control of eluant polarity. As the concentration of the organic modifier (normally methanol or acetonitrile) in the eluting buffer (mobile phase) is increased, it becomes less polar, and competes more effectively with the hydrophobic stationary phase. This decreases retention times for all compounds, having an effect on the chromatogram analogous to that of increased temperature in GLC.

More selective control of retention is available by altering the buffer pH. This alters the degree of ionisation of weak acids and bases, reduced ionisation being associated with increased retention. Reversed-phase packings are compatible with a pH range of about 2 to 8. The pK_a (dissociation constant) of the acid metabolites of the catecholamines (and indoleamines) lies within this range, and their retentions will all be increased as the pH drops over the range 4.5–2.5, and the equilibrium is shifted towards the un-ionised (and more hydrophobic) –COOH form. Parent catecholamines (and indoleamines) are, however, ionised ($-NH_3^+$ form) within the available pH range (and are anyway unstable at alkaline pH even if compatible columns were introduced). Control of their retention times can then be achieved by addition of an acidic ion-pairing agent (such as sodium octyl sulphate) to the running buffer. The precise mechanism of action of these compounds is still debated, but they have the effect of retarding postively charged molecules, the effect increasing with increasing alkyl chain length of the ion pairing agent.

Using spectrophotometric (UV) absorption detection, which has been the dominant mode of detection in HPLC, useful separations of a wide range of catecholamines (and indeed indoleamines) and metabolites can be demonstrated. However, the naturally occurring levels of biogenic amines and metabolites are near the limit of detection of UV, and UV is also not sufficiently selective. Thus a more sensitive and selective detection is necessary. From what has been said it is likely that indoles (including 5-hydroxy-indoles) would be suitable for detection by their native fluorescence, but that catechols will not be. Thus the extension of HPLC to naturally occurring levels of catecholamines and metabolites has depended on the development of a different mode of detection. The practical application of this mode of detection originated in the work of Professor R.N. Adams and his colleagues at Lawrence, Kansas, from the observation that catechols were among those compounds most readily oxidised at modest potentials at solid carbon electrodes. If a carbon paste or glassy carbon electrode is positioned in the effluent stream from an LC column and maintained at about +500 mV with respect to that flowing stream (this is achieved by the use of two further electrodes connected in the configuration familiar to electrophysiologists as voltage clamp), then compounds with the catechol group passing the electrode surface will be oxidised to the quinone form, giving up electrons to the positive 'working' electrode. These electrons can be detected as a small current, which is proportional to the catechol concentration at the electrode surface, and which can be converted to a potential and displayed on a conventional strip chart recorder. For any given setting of the working electrode potential, only compounds oxidising at or below the selected potential of the working electrode will be detected and hence measured. Oxidation potentials for a range of biogenic amines and related metabolites and precursors are given in Fig. 5.6. (There are of course a number of other more abundant constituents of biological materials, notably ascorbic and uric acids, which oxidise at similar potentials.) The resolving power of modern reversed-phase HPLC and the selectivity and sensitivity of electrochemical detection, which also requires an electrically conductive medium, are thus complementary in the use of HPLC-EC for assays of catecholamines and related compounds. 5-Hydroxyindoles oxidise at potentials only a little higher, and can also be detected. At about 0.7 V methylated catechols and indoles are detected, and at higher potentials phenols (including tyrosine) and indoles (including tryptophan) are detected. Recent reviews of the applications of electrochemical detection in the area of the biogenic amines are available (Kissinger *et al.*, 1981, and subsequent articles in *Life Sciences* **28**; Mefford, 1981; Marsden and Joseph, 1986).

5.4.3.2 *Apparatus*

(a) *Introduction.* The laboratory setting out to use HPLC is now faced with a bewildering choice of equipment ranging in price from less then £5000 to more than £20 000. All companies acknowledge that the essence of the separation is the column, when they want to sell columns. Manufacturers' prepacked columns cost between £100 and £200, clearly a small amount in relation to the total cost of the system. For anyone starting off to evaluate HPLC, I would recommend the purchase of modular equipment; that is, a pump, injection valve, column and detector as separate items. This gives maximum flexibility, and the range of analyses for which HPLC can be used is now so wide that it is virtually impossible that the equipment could become redundant. Figure 5.7 shows one such 'Heath Robinson' arrangement in our own laboratory. (See also Figs. 5.8, 5.14 and 5.15.)

On the other hand a laboratory may rightly be wary of taking on the business of 'plumbing up' separate components as well as all the other decisions that have to be made. In addition spare connectors, lengths of

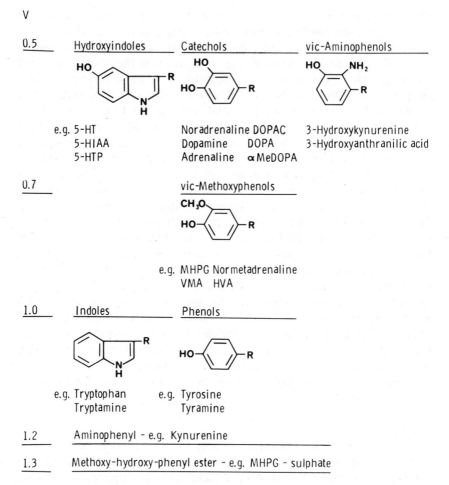

Fig. 5.6.   Approximate working potentials at which different chemical classes of compound are detected electrochemically.

tubing, etc. are unlikely to be available. A good compromise would appear to be a package of equipment that is set up but is inherently modular, such as the catecholamine analyser offered by Anachem. This gives a cheap introduction to HPLC, and all components can be upgraded subsequently, for example gradient elution (systematic variation of buffer composition during the separation) and, column temperature control, and belies its name by actually being useful for the full range of oxidative electrochemical assays.

If the laboratory already possesses HPLC equipment, then it is possible to add electrochemical detection in place of, or in series with, the existing

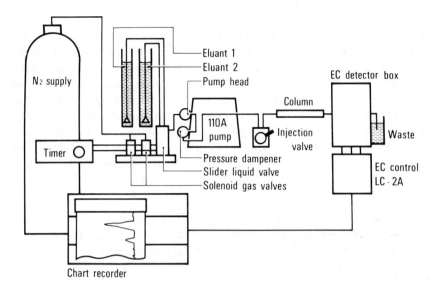

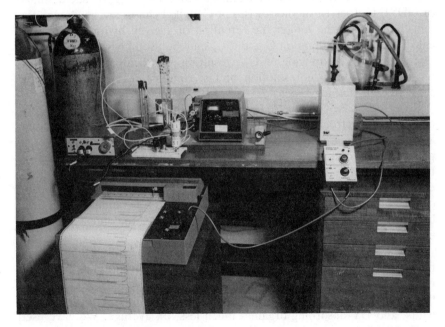

Fig. 5.7. HPLC system with EC detector and automatic step gradient facility. For detector details see Figs. 5.8 and 5.13.

detector. The advantages of serial detection, e.g. by fluorescence and electrochemistry, will be discussed later (section 5.5.2).

(b) *Columns and buffers.* Discussion here is confined to reversed-phase columns run with predominantly aqueous running buffers. A good review of available packings is given by Majors (1980). The best guide is to take a method from the literature and use it as a starting point. Bioanalytical Systems (BAS, West Lafayette, Indiana, USA, British agents Anachem Ltd, Luton; and Waters Instruments, British Agents Millipore UK, Harrow) publish a regularly updated bibliography of electrochemical methods. Batch-to-batch variation in packing is still a problem, and packings that are identical in specification from different manufacturers do behave differently for reasons that are not understood. Variables to consider are:

(i) *Particle size.* Finer packings will give higher resolution per unit length of column, but are of course more expensive and increase the working pressure for a given flow rate and column length. Suitable starting points are 10–15 cm columns of $5\mu m$ packing, or 25–30 cm columns of 10 μm packing.

(ii) *Alkyl chain length.* Silica packings bonded with C_{18} (octadecyl silane or ODS), C_8 (octyl), or shorter (C_2 or C_3) alkyl chains are available. The longer the chain the longer the retention of a given hydrophobic molecule. Most work is done on C_{18}, but C_8 may be useful where the range of retention times is too wide on C_{18}, resulting in difficulties in compromising between adequate resolution of fast running peaks and acceptably short overall running times.

Reversed-phase columns require relatively hydrophilic elution solvents, and since electrochemical detection requires a conducting medium, aqueous buffers are invariably a major component of the eluant. Column packings are compatible with a pH range of about 2–8. The concentration of the buffer species and its nature will affect the chromatography, e.g. phosphate gives greater retention than acetate. The exact proportion of organic modifier required will vary from column to column, even from batch to batch of a particular supplier's packing, and must be varied empirically in setting up the method.

Pure water is required for making up buffers, especially as the column filters many hundreds of litres of buffer during its life (unless solvent is recycled). However, purity requirements for EC detection will differ from those for UV detection; metal ions will be much more serious contaminants, and UV-absorbing organics much less, on average. We have used single distilled water successfully, and now use Millipore RQ purified water. 'Water for HPLC' is normally specifically cleaned up with UV detection in mind, but may be useful as a reference standard (see also notes on water purity for fluorescence analysis, section 5.3.4).

(c) *Electrochemical detectors.* Complete oxidation (coulometric detection) of the compounds detected will clearly give the most sensitive detection. However, the practical utility of a detector is governed by the signal-to-noise ratio, and as the noise level rises with the size of electrode and with turbulence in the flowing stream, there is no one simple answer to the problem of optimal detector-cell design. Also collection of fractions for further analysis after detection may imply limitations on dead volume and may make a small degree of oxidation desirable (as is obtained with amperometric detection).

The thin layer voltammetric flow cell design (Figure 5.8) which originated in Dr. Adams' laboratory (reviewed in Adams and Marsden (1982) and commercially available from BAS) undoubtedly made EC detection an extremely useful technique. Variants on this design include the provision of a glassy carbon auxiliary electrode opposite the working electrode, and positioning of the reference electrode in the working electrode block to reduce total dead volume. Other designs are increasingly appearing on the market offering a higher degree of substrate conversion (EDT, Metrohm, Kipp, ESA).

Electrode and cell material are also relevant considerations. The original working electrodes were carbon paste in mineral oil, packed into a cylindrical well in a perspex (plexiglass) block. Perspex has the advantage of being transparent so that bubbles are easily detected, but it is not resistent to high methanol or to any acetonitrile concentrations, and cells made of Kel-F are more versatile. Most authors feel that the oil-based carbon paste still offers the highest sensitivity in this design, and this is used where the ultimate in sensitivity is required, for example in plasma catecholamine determination. However, these electrodes do require repacking at intervals, the interval being markedly reduced by elevated organic modifier concentrations in the buffer. Accordingly other media for the carbon paste (silicone oil, paraffin wax) have been introduced. For routine use glassy carbon electrodes are to be preferred as they require very infrequent cleaning, which is simple to do, and have ample sensitivity for most applications.

(d) *Fluorescence detectors.* Although this topic is treated in section 5.5.2, some consideration of instrumentation is given here for continuity with the foregoing.

For a detector operating at fixed excitation and emission wavelengths over time, the requirements are different from those discussed in section 5.3.1 for an analytical instrument. A low-volume flow cell is used to

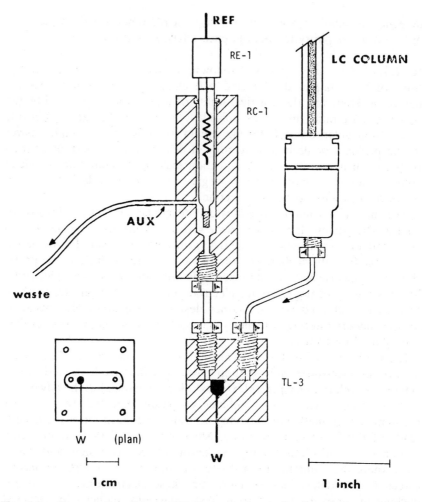

Fig. 5.8. Cross-section through TL-3 electrochemical cell, reference compartment and reference electrode. (TL-5 same as TL-3 but made of Kel-F and glassy carbon in place of plexiglass (perspex) and carbon paste.) Inset: plan view of Teflon spacer gasket (adapted from BAS LC-2A manual with permission).

prevent peak broadening, and the requirement is to get as much light into the sample as is practicable. Filter instruments, using a line source close to the excitation wavelength, permit a short path length. The specificity comes from the chromatography and not the fluorescence, thus a relatively broad band pass filter can be used for emission, again allowing a short light path. The Aminco Fluoromonitor is a cheap and suitable instrument, and modifications to enhance its performance have been described (Anderson *et al.*, 1979). The Kratos Schoeffel 950 is equally good value and better designed from the point of view of filter, lamp and flowcell accessibility. The considerably more expensive Schoeffel 970 is more sensitive and has continuously variable excitation wavelength. Where fluorescence detection is used alone (i.e. without electrochemical detection), stopped flow may be used to obtain spectra, but consideration of suitable scanning instruments falls outside the scope of this chapter.

5.4.3.3 *HPLC–EC determination of catecholamine metabolites*

(a) *General requirements for HPLC–EC.* Electrochemical detection requires a continuous flow of a conducting buffer past all three electrodes while the potential is applied to the working electrode. Bubbles due to decompression as the solvent emerges from the column are thus a particular problem, rather than just a source of noise as in other modes of detection. However, the degassing techniques used for HPLC in general are normally sufficient (ultrasonic bath, low pressure at the water pump or helium degassing). A degree of back-pressure across the detector, e.g. by using a long piece of relatively fine-bore tubing for the waste line, may help. We have used predominantly phosphate buffers with methanol as organic modifier. When high methanol concentrations are used, it is essential to ensure that the buffer species at the concentration used is soluble at this methanol concentration.

The buffer will then normally be taken up through a 2 μm filter by the pump and pumped at 1000–2000 psi (75–150 bar), through an injector on to the column. (The pressure is determined by the flow rate — we use 1 ml/min — and the column back-pressure.) A loop injector gives reproducible injection volumes (we use 20–200 μl), and should be equipped with a minimal dead volume syringe loading port so that where only small volumes of sample are available, they can be injected from a calibrated syringe. We normally operate the chromatograph with the injector in the 'inject' mode so that the sample loop is continuously flushed with solvent at high pressure. Switching smartly to the 'load' positions allows the loop to be filled at leisure and at atmospheric pressure, normally by injecting three or four loop volumes from a syringe. Smartly switching back to the 'inject' position delivers the sample on to the head of the column. We normally wash the column with 50% methanol:water before shutting down for the night, and running buffer flow must be re-established through the detector before the working electrode is switched on the next day. On switching on, the initial high current should decay to a steady background value. This will take anything from a few minutes to more than an hour, depending on the state of the electrode and the sensitivity at which it is to be used. If a high background current, or no deflection on switching on are observed, *do not leave the working electrode switched on.* The problem is usually due either to a bubble or faulty electrode connections. Carbon paste electrodes will also give a high background when they fail, i.e. when buffer establishes a direct path through the carbon paste to the metal contact electrode. They will then need repacking (do not wash the electrode well with water as this will facilitate subsequent failure).

(b) *Procedure.* Since acidic and neutral catecholamine (and indoleamine) metabolites are readily extracted from a deproteinised supernatant into an organic solution at acid pH, sample preparation is simple. Urine is acidified with HCl to ~0.5 N, (pH < 1) (after previous hydrolysis of conjugates if required — see section 5.4.2.1), and extracted twice with ethyl acetate. Solvent is removed from the combined extracts by a gentle stream of nitrogen, and the sample is reconstituted in the starting volume of distilled water or running buffer. In our method (Joseph *et al.*, 1981b) we use a 0.1 M phosphate buffer pH 3 containing 5 to 15% methanol, and a 15 or 25 cm column of Shandon Hypersil ODS 5 μm. Injection volume is 20 μl using a syringe-loading loop injector. In this way we can resolve VMA, MHPG, DOPAC, 5-HIAA and HVA, with electrochemical detection at a sensitivity of 50–100 nA/V and a potential of 0.7 V (Fig. 5.9) (0.5 V will detect only the non-methylated metabolites (DOPAC, 5-HIAA)). We circumvented the problem of combining adequate resolution of fast running peaks with an acceptable overall running time by using step gradient elution, the elution buffer being automatically switched at the pump inlet from 5% methanol to 15% methanol 5.5 min after the start of the run. This front reaches the detector 8 min later. This device (Fig. 5.7) is a very cheap (~ £250) alternative to upgrading a single pump to full gradient facility (£2500 to £5500). However, subsequent availability of gradient equipment has resolved further peaks in urine samples. In particular a large peak close to DOPAC may interfere in the method as published. It is still suitable for clinical chemistry screening, but we have introduced the following modifications for psychopharmacological use:

Column: — Altex Ultraspheres column 15 × 0.45 cm. ODS 5 μm with a 2.5 × 0.45 cm guard column.
Buffer: — A = 0.1 M sodium phosphate pH 2.6, 0.01% EDTA;
B = 0.1 M sodium phosphate pH 3.5, 0.01% EDTA, 30% methanol.
Gradient: — 7% B (10 min); 7 to 50% B (30 min); 50 to 100% B (20 min); 100% B (hold 25 min); 100 to 7% B (5 min); 7% B (hold 10 min before next injection).

Figure 5.10 shows a trace from a urine sample processed and run in this way (a), and from the same sample spiked before analysis with added standards (b).

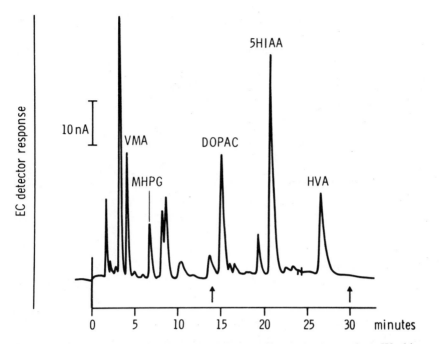

Fig. 5.9. HPLC–EC analysis of amine metabolites in human urine. Working potential 0.72 V. Arrows indicate switch from 5 to 15% methanol and 15 to 5% methanol (reaching detector) in 0.1M phosphate buffer, pH 3.0. (From Joseph *et al.*, 1981b.)

Exactly the same principles are applicable to primate brain tissue (Cross and Joseph, 1981). Protein can be precipitated at pH 3 with a citrate/phosphate buffer, and the acid and neutral metabolites extracted directly into ethyl acetate from the supernatant. Here VMA is present in very low concentration, and MHPG, DOPAC, 5-HIAA and HVA can be resolved with an isocratic buffer: 0.1 M phosphate pH 4.0 and 10% methanol (Fig. 5.11). In rat brain MHPG is predominantly in the conjugated form and hence will not be determined without prior hydrolysis.

In CSF appreciable amounts of the amines are not present, and thus HPLC of the native CSF can be carried out directly. In this way we can resolve MHPG (in humans), 5-HIAA and HVA (Baker *et al.*, 1980; Joseph *et al.*, 1981a). (Fig. 5.12) We normally filter CSF before direct injection (Joseph *et al.*, 1981c — see section 5.2.1.3) in order to ensure removal of protein, particulate matter and any potentially infectious agents.

5.4.3.4 *HPLC-EC assay of catecholamines.* As previously described, amines can be retained more effectively on the column by addition of

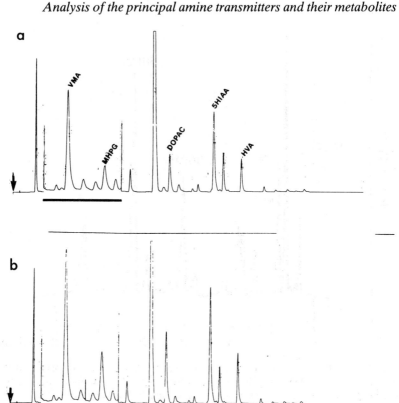

Fig. 5.10.   Gradient HPLC–EC analysis of amine metabolites in human urine (a)
Hydrolysed urine sample. Conditions as in text. Peaks identified by spiking with
authentic standards (shown in (b)). Chart speed increased two-fold and detector
amplification increased eight fold from 8 to 33 min (underlined). Total run time
75 min.

ion-pairing agents to the buffer. Since noradrenaline in particular elutes
rather rapidly at even low methanol concentrations, this is the approach
adopted by most published methods (see 'Current Concepts' *Life Sciences*
(2 February 1981) following the reference to Kissinger *et al.*, 1981; also
Marsden and Joseph, 1986). The effectiveness of an alkyl sulphate or
alkyl sulphonate in retarding amines will increase with alkyl chain length
and also with concentration, up to a maximum usually in the 5 mM
region. Longer alkyl chain length on the other hand will result in slower
equilibration of the buffer with the column. Thus for any particular
separation an appropriate alkyl chain length of ion-pairing agent, and
indeed of column packing, is sought.
    Prior separation of the catecholamines from other metabolites is often
achieved using adsorption on to alumina at neutral pH and recovery at

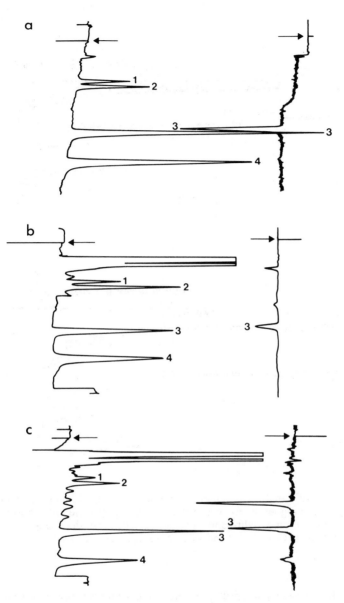

Fig. 5.11. HPLC determination, with dual detection, of amine metabolites in human brain.

Electrochemical (Lt) and fluorescence (Rt) detector traces from chromatography as described in text, of (a) standard mixture: 1, MHPG (2 ng); 2, DOPAC (2 ng); 3, 5-HIAA (10 ng); 4 HVA (10 ng); and of extracts of (b) human hypothalamus; (c) human temporal cortex (equivalent of 40 mg each applied to the column). Arrows indicate injection of 200 μl samples. Full-scale deflection = 20nA EC (reduced to 100nA for peaks b 3, 4); 16 mV fluorescent (reduced to 160 mV for B).

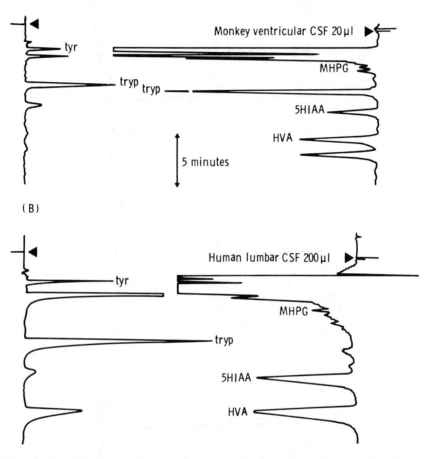

Fig. 5.12. HPLC analysis of amine metabolites in filtered untreated primate CSF. (A) Cynomolgous monkey ventricular CSF. Left-hand side: fluorescence detection 254/330 nm; right-hand side: electrochemical detection, $V = 1.0$. (B) Human lumbar CSF. Left-hand side: as above; right-hand side: as above, but $V = 0.7$.

acid pH. In this way catechols (i.e. the catecholamines and precursor and metabolites that retain the catechol grouping (DOPA, DHPG, DOPAC)) are separated from methylated metabolites (MHPG, VMA, HVA) and the metadrenalines, and 5-hydroxyindoles (5-HT, 5-HIAA). This is mandatory for the assay of low levels of catecholamines found in urine or the even lower levels in plasma (Falconer *et al.*, 1982; Marsden and Joseph, 1986). In tissues such as brain where catecholamines are more abundant, it is possible to assay the total protein-free supernatant by utilising selective detection rather than prior extraction; by setting the electrochemical detector at a suitable voltage (~0.5 V), methylated metabolites are not detected. 5-Hydroxyindoles are detected, but a relatively high pH will bring DOPAC and 5-HIAA off early and the ion-pair agent concentration can be adjusted to avoid interference with noradrenaline, the fastest running of the amines. The remaining problem is the long retention of 5-HT relative to NA and DA; this can be dealt with by injecting samples at intervals such that the 5-HT peak comes off with the chromatogram of the next sample. A more elegant solution is to exploit selective effects of different organic modifiers (Mayer and Shoup, 1983), or pairing agents with a gradient of methanol (Joseph, 1985).

5.4.3.5 *Trouble shooting*. Problems with the electrochemical detector normally take the form of a background current or noise level which is too high, or a sensitivity which is too low. Many problems in the system can be traced to air bubbles either running through the cell (result: glitches — sharp increases and/or decreases of signal followed by return to baseline), or stationary between electrodes (result: high or zero background) or at some other point (result: amplification of pump pressure pulsations leading to regular baseline oscillations). More exhaustive degassing of the eluant buffer may be required by a combination of the previously mentioned methods, e.g. low pressure with ultrasonic degassing. With gradient work, when low and high concentrations of organic modifier are being mixed in varying proportions, gas bubbles may be expelled only during one part of the gradient, especially if buffer reservoir temperatures vary during the day. Continuous degassing with a slow flow of helium has been found to be effective in this case.

Another source of high background current is metal ions from the HP tubing or pump dissolving in the mobile phase. This can be ameliorated by avoiding buffers containing chloride ions, and by including EDTA (at say 0.01%) in the running buffer. Passifying metal components (but not the packed column) by pumping 6M nitric acid is recommended by some manufacturers. In our early experiments with solvent switching and gradient work we obtained large humps in the baseline when switching from one solvent or pump to another. This has led many authors to conclude that EC cannot be used with solvent switching or programming. In fact we were able to trace these problems to metal ions from the solvent inlet filters (in which the solvent is exposed to a large surface area of metal) or pump chamber, connecting tubing or damping coil building up in the solvent in the stationary part of the system to a level higher than that in the flowing part. A combination of replacing metal inlet filters with sintered glass, addition of EDTA to the buffers and/or rearranging plumbing resolved these problems.

Too low a sensitivity of the electrode is usually due to poisoning of the surface, which will involve repacking a carbon paste electrode, or polishing (e.g. with alumina paste) a glassy carbon one. The other major source of noise is electrical interference. The waste outlet should flow into and not drip into the waste beaker, and the instrument should be situated well away from, and with a mains supply well away from, the mains supply to heavy equipment such as centrifuges and scintillation counters. For very sensitive work, copper mesh Faraday cages are used to shield the detector or the whole instrument. Good earthing is also essential, as is the avoidance of earth loops. Nonetheless most modern EC detectors will work quite well when just placed on the bench, connected to the system and switched on.

The other source of problems is the column. Some compounds do not chromatograph well on some suppliers' packings for reasons that are poorly understood. Other than trying the effect of ion-pair reagents or other additives to improve peak tailing, it is usually a matter of trial and error to match separations, column and buffer. As with other forms of HPLC, peak broadening will result from excessive dead volumes between injector and column and between column and detector. Tubing runs should be of minimum practicable length and bore (0.3 mm i.d. or less).

Distortions in peak shape developing over time as samples are run (asymmetry or even peak splitting, when seen for all the peaks observed) are nearly always due to settling of the packed column bed leaving asymmetrical voids below the entry frit (filter). This can be cured by levelling the top of the column and repacking with a paste of the same packing in methanol, or with glass beads so that no gap is left. Both this procedure and a clean-up washing cycle for contaminated columns, the other source of peak distortion, are well reviewed by Rabel (1980). (See also notes on solvents and reagents, and on the effects of concentration from relatively large volumes in section 5.3.4.)

5.5 Synthesis of approaches

5.5.1 *Separation of classes of compound*
From what has been said in the previous section, it is clear that HPLC with electrochemical detection can in principle separate all catecholamines and indole amines and their metabolites in a single run. While this has been reported by some authors (Van Valkenburg *et al.*, 1982; Wagner *et al.*, 1982), problems arise where determination of a disproportionately minor component is required. In such a case prior separation is required, often into classes of compounds, e.g. amines/acidic metabolites/neutral metabolites or catechols/noncatechols. It is often more practical to do this than to try to resolve all amines and metabolites at once. It becomes more difficult to find a compromise giving good resolution and peak

shape, without inordinately long retention times for any compound, as the number of components increases. Thus fractions from standard column procedures for amine and metabolite separations (Atack, 1977; Westerink and Korf, 1977) can be analysed by HPLC (e.g. Westerink and Mulder, 1981). The procedure described in section 5.3.3 will also give fractions suitable for HPLC (Curzon *et al.*, 1981), the final neutral extract containing acid metabolites and the organic phase neutral metabolites. The acid phase contains amines and amino acids, which can then be separated by the supplementary procedure described here (section 5.3.3).

5.5.2 *HPLC with fluorescence detection*
5.5.2.1 *Introduction.* From what has been said in section 5.3.1 on native fluorescence of indoles (which is shared by 5-hydroxyindoles) it is clear that they are good candidates for fluorescence detection. Of the amines, precursors and metabolites present in the tissues we have considered, only tyrosine, other than the indoles and 5-hydroxyindoles, is present in large enough amounts to contribute to the fluorescence at the indole optimum of 280/330 nm. The practical result of this is that fluorescence detection at these wavelengths is *more* selective than electrochemical detection, although it is difficult to achieve the same sensitivity. Thus where only the 5-hydroxyindole pathway is to be studied, fluorescence detection may be preferred to electrochemical.

Whole blood 5-HT can be estimated on a deproteinised extract (see section 5.2.1.2 (b)) by fluorescence (Joseph, 1978a, and section 5.3.1). The same extract can be analysed by HPLC with fluorescence detection. We use 10% methanol in 0.1 M NaH_2PO_4 on Hypersil ODS 5. Peaks are seen for tyrosine, 5-HTP (if present), 5-HT, tryptophan and 5-HIAA (if present) (Fig. 5.13). However, recovery (other than that of 5-HT) may be poor and/or unreliable.

Plasma determinations of 5-hydroxyindoles are required in studies using 5-HTP administration, and for screening for carcinoid syndrome. Simple methanol deproteinisation of plasma (4 volumes MeOH) and dilution back to 10% MeOH with 0.1 M NaH_2PO_4 gives an extract suitable for direct injection for HPLC analysis of tyrosine, 5-HTP, 5-HT (N.B. plasma levels very low, since nearly all whole blood 5-HT is in platelets), tryptophan, 5-HIAA and 5-hydroxytryptophol (if present). Determination of CSF 5-HIAA is discussed below. Instrumentation has been discussed in section 5.4.3.2(d).

5.5.2.2 *Dual detection.* The complementary specificities of fluorescent and electrochemical detection, especially since the EC detection threshold is so readily adjusted, make the use of both detectors in series particularly attractive. This is borne out in results presented by Anderson

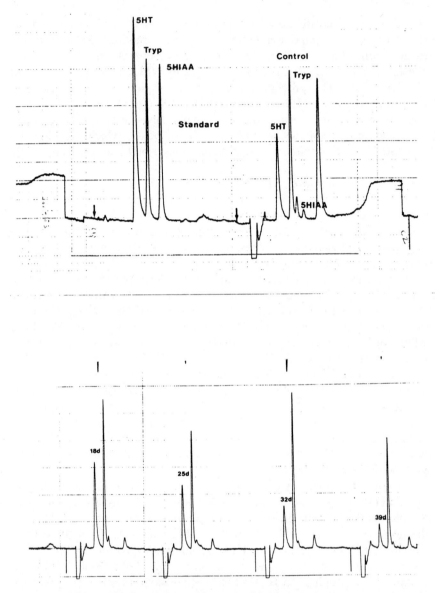

Fig. 5.13.   HPLC–F analysis of whole blood (platelet) 5-HT. (a) 5-HT, trypto-phan, 5-HIAA mixed standard, 100 ng/ml; (b) control blood sample (infant); (c) the effect of fenfluramine treatment, 25–30 mg/day given from day 14 to day 39 of trial, on whole blood 5-HT in a 6-year-old autistic child.

et al. (1979) as well as by ourselves (Cross and Joseph, 1981; Joseph *et al.*, 1981a; Joseph and Davies, 1983).

Figure 5.14 depicts an isocratic (single-solvent) system with fluorescence and electrochemical detectors arranged in series. With the large dead volume contained in the reference compartment with this design of flow cell (TL-5; Figs. 5.8 and 5.15) it is mandatory that the fluorescent detector be upstream of the EC detector, and that the two are connected by fine-bore tubing. In the TL-7 or TL-8 detector cell from BAS the reference electrode screws directly into the working electrode compartment, reducing the total dead volume for subsequent fraction collection. Even this detector, however, is better placed downstream of a fluorescence detector, since problems may arise from the conversion of metabolites into oxidised products at the working electrode (about 5% of total with this type of detector).

For compounds giving peaks on both detectors (indoles, 5-hydroxyindoles, tyrosine) peak ratios can provide a routine check that other substances are not co-eluting. This is particularly useful in dealing with human clinical samples with the possibility of drug metabolites or other idiosyncratic interferences. If enough material is available, repeat runs at different electrode potentials can give even more positive identification. An obvious improvement would be to obtain this information on a single run using multiple electrodes. However, because of the way in which the working electrode potential is controlled, two single electrode detector cells each with its own control box cannot simply be placed in series and set to different potentials. Double electrode control boxes following the principles described by Blank (1976) are now commercially available, and some applications using simultaneous or sequential detection at different potentials have been described (Mayer and Shoup, 1983; Langlais *et al.*, 1984; Marsden and Joseph, 1986).

Compounds present in very different concentrations can be more satisfactorily dealt with using dual detection. Thus in human lumbar CSF, MHPG is present in rather small quantities (*c.* 10 ng/g), 5-HIAA is at about 25 ng/g, but tryptophan is present at some 300 ng/g. If the EC detector is operated at 1.0 V to determine tryptophan, 5-HIAA appears as a peak on its tail. By setting the EC detector to 0.7 V, tryptophan is virtually undetected, but can still be quantified on the fluorescence detector (Fig. 5.12B). Tyrosine, present in even larger amounts, will also not be detected at this potential (in fact it is not retained enough to be separated from the solvent front on the EC detector anyway), but is clearly resolved on the more selective fluorescence detector.

Figure 5.16 illustrates again the separation of the indoles 5-HTP, 5-HT, tryptophan and 5-HIAA with dual detection (compare Fig. 5.13). All

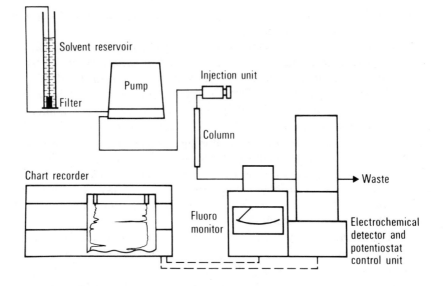

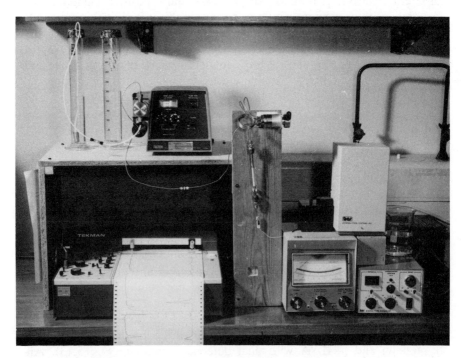

Fig. 5.14.   HPLC system: isocratic with fluorescence and EC detection in series.

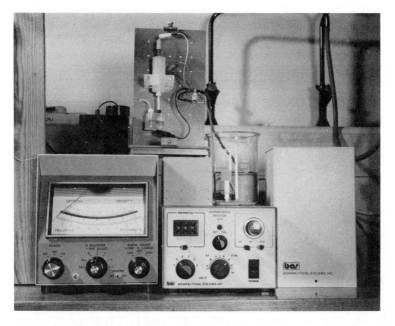

Fig. 5.15. Detail of detectors from Fig. 5.14. (For EC detector cf. Fig. 5.8.)

four are seen on the fluorescence detector, but tryptophan is virtually undetected on the electrochemical detector operating at 0.7 V.

5.5.3 *Conclusion: the use of multiple assays*

Much of the progress in the understanding of the role of the biogenic amines in the response to drugs and in normal and abnormal behaviour has depended upon reliable assays for amines, precursors and metabolites. However, our ideas on which system subserves which function have often been shaped by looking only at the system that was expected to be responsible, and often, even today, at only one component of that system, e.g. one amine or one metabolite. Even at this level, the simplification of work-up procedures and degree of identification at the detection stage would give HPLC a major advantage over many other procedures employed.

The development of HPLC for these multiple assays, however, parallels a developing awareness among psychopharmacologists of the importance of studying interactions between one aminergic system and another (and indeed between aminergic and non-aminergic systems) in understanding evolving drug actions and their behavioural effects. A great advantage of HPLC methods is that you may see a change in the system you did not expect to change as well as, or instead of, in the one you did.

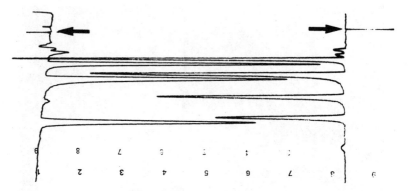

Fig. 5. 16.   Isocratic resolution of indole standards. Left-hand side EC detection, V = 0.7. Right-hand side: fluorescence detection 254/330 nm; peaks in order of eleation: 1, 5-HTP; 2, 5-HT; 3, tryptophan; 4, 5-HIAA.

5.6 **Postscript**

5.6.1 *Amino acids*

I have already mentioned that HPLC-EC and HPLC-F can be applied to the determination of the amino acid precursors of the biogenic amines. These include tryptophan and tyrosine, which are also constituents of protein. The majority of other protein constituent amino acids do not have useful native fluorescence or electrochemical activity. This includes the putative neurotransmitter amino acids, glutamate, aspartate, glycine and also γ-amino butyric acid (GABA) and taurine, omega amino acids which are particularly abundant in nervous tissue. However, all primary amino acids will react with *o*-phthalaldehyde/mercaptoethanol reagent under alkaline conditions (pH 9, 2 min, room temperature) to yield fluorescent isoindoles. The OPT–ME products chromatograph well on reversed-phase systems of the type described earlier, at somewhat higher methanol concentrations (Lindroth and Mopper, 1979; Jones *et al.*, 1981). Small peptides behave similarly, and the OPT–ME derivatives of both amino acids and peptides are electrochemically active (Joseph and Davies, 1983; Joseph and Marsden, 1986). Thus HPLC-EC and HPLC-F show great promise for studying the chemistry of other classes of trans-mitters and in turn their interactions with the amine systems.

5.6.2 *In vivo detection of amines*

Although measurements of amines and metabolites in small areas of brain tissue are unquestionably useful, they do not allow distinction between inactive intracellular pools and active or ex-active extracellular pools of amines and metabolites. The same principle used to detect amines emerging from the HPLC column can be applied to amines being released in specific areas of the brain of conscious unrestrained animals. Working microelectrodes of carbon paste or carbon fibre are stereotactically implanted along with miniature reference and auxiliary electrodes (Marsden, 1984; Kennett and Joseph, 1982; Hutson and Curzon, 1983; O'Neill *et al.*, 1983; Joseph *et al.*, 1986). No chromatographic identification of the species present is occurring, but a degree of electrochemical identification is possible by applying a ramp potential to the electrode, and observing the half-wave oxidation potential. (This contrasts with the fixed potential used for EC detection in HPLC, where the flow of solvent results in a continually changing concentration at the working electrode.) This represents a further application of electrochemical technique in the study of brain amine systems, which complements *ex-vivo* analysis in a completely new way.

Acknowledgements

I will not exhaust the reader, or myself, by attempting to list all the colleagues who have contributed to the development of these methods. I would like to thank all the staff of the Division of Psychiatry, especially Dennis Risby, Harry Baker, Alan Cross and Frank Owen, and my students David Hall-Tipping, Bas Kadam, Guy Kennett and Phillip Davies.

Particular thanks are also due to Richard Green and Gerald Curzon for introducing me to the fluorescence techniques, and to Don Walter and Sandy Pullar for GLC techniques. In the HPLC field I must thank Dr. Chung-Ki Lim for introduction and continuing advice, and Ralph Adams, Charles Marsden, Simon Young and George Anderson for continuing discussions and advice.

References to equipment from particular manufacturers are included as examples; no denigration of other commercially available equipment is intended or implied.

References

Adams, R.N. and Marsden, C.A. (1982). Electrochemical detection methods for monoamine measurements *in vitro* and *in vivo*. In *Handbook of Psychopharmacology*, vol. 15. (L.L. Iversen, S.D. Iversen and S.H. Snyder, Eds), 1–74, Plenum, New York.

Anderson, G.M., Young, J.G. and Cohen, D.J. (1979). Rapid liquid chromatographic determination of tryptophan, tyrosine, 5HIAA and HVA in CSF. *J. Chromatog.* **164**, 501–5.

Atack, C. (1977). Measurement of biogenic amines using cation exchange chromatography and fluorimetric assay. *Acta Physiol. Scand. (Suppl.)* **451**, 1–99.

Baker, C.A. and Johnson, G.A. (1981). Radioenzymic assay of dihydroxyphenylglycol (DOPEG) and dihydroxyphenylethanol (DOPET) in plasma and cerebrospinal fluid. *Life Sci.* **29**, 165–72.

Baker, H.F., Joseph, M.H. and Ridley, R.M. (1980). HPLC analysis of tryptophan, 5HIAA and HVA using fluorescence and EC detection; the effect of probenecid studied in primate ventricular CSF. *Brit. J. Pharmacol.* **70**, 133P–4P.

Blanchard, J. (1981). Evaluation of the relative efficiency of various techniques for deproteinising plasma samples prior to HPLC analysis. *J. Chromatog.* **226**, 455–60.

Blank, C.L. (1976). Dual electrochemical detector for liquid chromatography. *J. Chromatog.* **117**, 35–46.

Blomberry, P.A., Kopin, I.J., Gordon, E.K., Markey, S.P. and Ebert, M.H. (1980). Conversion of MHPG to vanillylmandelic acid; implications for the importance of urinary MHPG. *Arch. Gen. Psychiat.* **37**, 1095–8.

Chang, C.C. (1964). A sensitive method for spectrophotometric assay of catecholamines. *Int. J. Neuropharmac.* **3**, 643–9.

Coyle, J.T. and Henry, D. (1973). Catecholamines in foetal and newborn rat brain. *J. Neurochem.* **21**, 61–7.

Cross, A.J. and Joseph, M.H. (1981). The concurrent estimation of the major monoamine metabolites in human and non-human primate brain by HPLC with fluorescence and electrochemical detection. *Life Sci.* **28**, 499–505.

Curzon, G. and Green, A.R. (1970). Rapid method for the determination of 5-hydroxytryptamine and 5-hydroxyindoleacetic acid in small regions of rat brain. *Brit. J. Pharmacol.* **39**, 653–5.

Curzon, G., Kantamaneni, B.D. and Tricklebank, M.D. (1981). A comparison of an improved OPT fluorometric method and HPLC in the determination of brain 5-hydroxyindoles of rats treated with L-tryptophan and p-chlorophenylalanine. *Brit. J. Pharmacol.* **73**, 555–61.

De Met, E.M. and Halaris, A.E. (1979). Origin and distribution of 3-methoxy-4-hydroxyphenylglycol in body fluids. *Biochem. Pharmacol.* **28**, 3043–50.

Dekirmenjian, H. and Maas, J.W. (1970). An improved procedure of 3-methoxy-4-hydroxyphenylethylene glycol determination by GLC. *Anal. Biochem.* **35**, 113–22.

Duggan, D.E. and Udenfriend, S. (1956). The spectrophotofluorometric detemination of tryptophan in plasma and of tryptophan and tyrosine in protein hydrolysates. *J. Biol. Chem.* **223**, 313–19.

Falconer, A.D., Lake, D. and Macdonald, I.A. (1982). The measurement of plasma noradrenaline by HPLC with electrochemical detection: an assessment of sample stability and assay reproducibility. *J. Neurosci. Meth.*, **6**, 261–71.

Fawcett, J., Maas, J.W. and Dekirmenjian, H. (1972). Depression and MHPG excretion. *Arch. Gen. Psychiat.* **26**, 246–51.

Geeraerts, F., Schimpfessel, L. and Crokaert, R. (1974). A simple routine method to preserve and determine blood serotonin. *Experientia* **30**, 837.

Holly, J.M.P. and Makin, H.L.J. (1983). The estimation of catecholamines in human plasma. *Anal. Biochem.* **128**, 257–74.

Hutson, P.H. and Curzon, G. (1983). Monitoring *in vivo* of transmitter metabolism by electrochemical methods. *Biochem. J.* **211**, 1–12.

Jones, B.N., Paabo, S. and Stein, S. (1981). Amino acid analysis and enzymic sequence determination of peptides by an improved *o*-phthaldialdehyde precolumn labelling procedure. *J. Liq. Chromatog.* **4**, 565–86.

Joseph, M.H. (1978a). Brain tryptophan metabolism on the 5-hydroxytryptamine and kynurenine pathways in a strain of rats with a deficiency in platelet 5HT. *Brit. J. Pharmacol.* **63**, 529–33.

Joseph, M.H. (1978b). The determination of kynurenine; a simple GLC method applicable to urine, plasma, brain and CSF. *J. Chromatog. (Biomed. Applicns)* **146**, 33–41.

Joseph, M.H. (1985). Alkyl-boronates as catechol-specific mobile phase pairing agents; application to HPLC analysis of biogenic amines, precursors and metabolites in brain tissue. *J. Chromatog. (Biomed. Applicns)* **342**, 370–75.

Joseph, M.H. and Baker, H.F. (1976). The determination of 5-hydroxy-tryptophan and its metabolites in plasma following administration to man. *Clin. Chim. Acta.* **72**, 125–31.

Joseph, M.H. and Davies, P. (1983). The electrochemical activity of OPT-amino acides; application to HPLC determination of amino acids in plasma and other biological materials. *J. Chromatog.* **277**, 125–36.

Joseph, M.H. and Deakin, J.F.W. (1977). *Biochemistry of Transmitters in the Brain*, E.R. Squibb and Sons, Twickenham, Middlesex.

Joseph, M.H. and Halliday, J. (1975). A dansylation microassay for some amino acids in brain. *Anal. Biochem.* **64**, 389–402.

Joseph, M.H. and Marsden, C.A. (1986). Amino acids and small peptides. In *HPLC of small molecules* (C.K. Lim, Ed), IRL, Oxford, *in press*.

Joseph, M.H., Baker, H.F., Crow, T.J. and Johnstone, E.C. (1976). Determination of 3-methoxy-4-hydroxyphenylglycol conjugates in urine; application to schizophrenic patients. *Psychopharmacology* **51**, 47–51.

Joseph, M.H., Baker, H.F., Johnstone, E.C. and Crow, T.J. (1979). MHPG excretion in acutely schizophrenic patients during a controlled clinical trial of the isomers of flupenthixol. *Psychopharmacology* **64**, 35–40.

Joseph, M.H., Baker, H.F. and Ridley, R.M. (1981a). Analysis of CSF amine metabolites and precursors including tryptophan, 5HIAA and HVA by HPLC using fluorescence and electrochemical detection; the effects of probenecid studied in primates. In *Central Neurotransmitter Turnover* (C. Pycock and P. Taberner, Eds), 162–7, Croom Helm, London.

Joseph, M.H., Fillenz, M., Macdonald, I.A. and Marsden, C.A. (Eds) (1986). *Monitoring neurotransmitter release during behaviour,* VCH/Ellis Horwood, Chichester.

Joseph, M.H., Kadam, B.V. and Risby, D. (1981b). Simple HPLC method for the concurrent determination of the amine metabolites VMA, MHPG, 5HIAA, DOPAC and HVA in urine using electrochemical detection. *J. Chromatog.* **226**, 361–8.

Joseph, M.H., Kadam, B.V. and Sanders, D. (1981c). A simple device using disposable tubes for ultrafiltration of small samples for protein binding studies. *Lab. Practice* **30**, 348–9.

Joseph, M.H., Owen, F., Baker, H.F. and Bourne, R.C. (1977), Platelet seroto-nin concentration and monoamine oxidase activity in unmedicated chronic schizophrenic and in schizoaffective patients. *Psychol. Med.* **7**, 159–62.

Kennett, G.A. and Joseph, M.H. (1982). Does *in vivo* voltammetry in the hippocampus measure 5HT release? *Brain Res.* **236**, 305–16.

Kissinger, P.T., Bruntlett, C.S. and Shoup, R.E. (1981). Neurochemical applications of liquid chromatography with electrochemical detection. *Life Sci.* **28**, 455–65.

Korf, J. and Valkenburgh-Sikkema, T. (1969). Fluorimetric determination of 5HIAA in human urine and CSF. *Clin. Chim. Acta* **26**, 301–6.

Langlais, P.J., Bird, E.D. and Matson, W.R. (1984). An automated HPLC, three-cell electrochemical method for the simultaneous assay of monoamines and metabolites in crude brain extracts. *Clin. Chem.*, **30**, 1047. (See also Matson, W.R. *et al.*, *ibid*, 1477–88.)

Lindroth, P. and Mopper, K. (1979). HPLC determination of subpicomole amounts of amino acids by precolumn fluorescence derivatization with *o-*

phthaldialdehyde. *Anal. Chem.* **51** 1667–74.

Maas, J.W., Hattox, S.E., Greene, N.M. and Landis, D.H. (1979). 3-methoxy-4-hydroxyphenethyleneglycol production by human brain *in vivo*. *Science* **205**, 1025–7.

Maickel, R.P. and Miller, F.P. (1966). Fluorescent products formed by reaction of indole derivatives and *o*-phthalaldehyde. *Anal. Chem.* **38**, 1937–8.

Majors, R.E. (1980). Recent advances in HPLC packings and columns. *J. Chrom. Sci.* **18**, 488–511.

Mardh, G., Sjoquist, B. and Anggard, E. (1981). Norepinephrine metabolism in man using deuterium labelling: the conversion of 4-hydroxy-3-methoxyphenylglycol to 4-hydroxy-3-methoxymandelic acid. *J. Neurochem.* **36**, 1181–85.

Mardh, G., Sjoquist, B. and Anggard, E. (1983). Norepinephrine metabolism in humans studied by deuterium labelling: turnover of 4-hydroxy-3-methoxyphenylglycol. *J. Neurochem.*, **41**, 246–50.

Marsden, C.A. (1984). (Ed) *Measurement of neurotransmitter release in vivo*. IBRO/John Wiley, Chichester.

Marsden, C.A. and Joseph, M.H. (1986). Biogenic amines *In HPLC of small molecules* (C.K. Lim, Ed), IRL, Oxford, *in press*.

Mayer, G.S. and Shoup, R.E. (1983). Simultaneous multiple electrode liquid chromatographic–electrochemical assay for catecholamines, indoleamines and metabolites in brain tissue. *J. Chromatog.*, **255**, 533–44.

Meek, J.L. and Neff. N.H. (1972). Fluorometric estimation of HMPG-sulphate in brain. *Brit. J. Pharmacol.* **45**, 435–41.

Mefford, I.N. (1981). Application of HPLC with EC detection to neurochemical analysis: measurement of catecholamines, serotonin and metabolites in rat brain. *J. Neurosci. Meth.* **3**, 207–24.

Murphy, G.F., Robinson, D. and Sharman, D.F. (1969). The effect of tropolone on the formation of 3,4-dihydroxyphenylacetic acid and 4-hydroxy-3-methoxyphenylacetic acid in the brain of the mouse. *Brit. J. Pharmacol.* **36**, 107–15.

Muscettola, G., Potter, W.Z., Gordon, E.K. and Goodwin, F.K. (1981). Methodological issues in the measurement of urinary MHPG. *Psychiat. Res.* **4**, 267–76.

O'Neill, R.D., Fillenz, M. and Albery, W.J. (1983). The development of linear sweep voltammetry with carbon paste electrodes *in vivo*. *J. Neurosci, Meth.* **8**, 263–73.

Rabel, F.M. (1980). Use and maintenance of microparticle HPLC columns. *J. Chromatog. Sci.* **18**, 394–408.

Rodnight, R. (1975). Obtaining, fixing and extracting neural tissues. In *Practical Neurochemistry* (H. McIlwain, Ed.), 2nd Edn, 1–16, Churchill Livingstone, Edinburgh.

Saller, C.F. and Zigmond, M.J. (1978). A radioenzymic assay for catecholamines and dihydroxyphenylacetic acid. *Life Sci.* **23**, 1117–30.

Snyder, S.H., Axelrod, J. and Zweig, M. (1965). A sensitive and specific fluorescence assay for tissue serotonin. *Biochem. Pharmacol.* **14**, 831–5.

Udenfriend, S. (1962, 1969). *Fluorescence Assay in Biology and Medicine*, Vols 1 and 2, Academic Press, New York.

Udenfriend, S., Titus, E. and Weissbach, H. (1955). The identification of 5-hydroxy-3-indoleacetic acid in normal urine and a method for its assay. *J. Biol. Chem.* **216**, 499–505.

Udenfriend, S., Weissbach, H. and Brodie, B.B. (1958). Assay of serotonin and related metabolites, enzymes and drugs. *Meth. Biochem. Anal.* **6**, 112–13.

Van Valkenburg, C.F.M., Tjaden, U.R., van der Krogt, J.A. and van der Leden, A. (1982). Determination of dopamine and its acid metabolites in brain tissue by HPLC with electrochemical detection in a single run after minimal sample pretreatment. *J. Neurochem.* **39**, 990–7.

Vanable, J.W. Jr (1963). A ninhydrin reaction giving a sensitive quantitative fluorescence assay for 5-hydroxytryptamine. *Anal. Biochem.* **6**, 393–403.

Wagner, J., Vitali, P., Palfreyman, M.G., Zraika, M. and Huot, S. (1982). Simultaneous determination of DOPA, 5HTP, dopamine, 3 O-Me DOPA, noradrenaline, DOPAC, HVA, 5HT, and 5HIAA in rat CSF and brain by HPLC with electrochemical detection. *J. Neurochem.* **38**, 1241–54.

Walter, D.S. and Shilcock, G.M. (1977). Urinary MHPG, an index of peripheral rather than central adrenergic activity in the rat. *J. Pharm. Pharmac.* **29**, 626–7.

Westerink, B.H.C. and Korf, J. (1977). Rapid concurrent automated fluorimetric assay of noradrenaline, dopamine, DOPAC, HVA and 3-methoxytyramine in milligram amounts of nervous tissue after isolation on Sephadex G10. *J. Neurochem.* **29**, 697–706.

Westerink, B.H.C. and Mulder, T.B.A. (1981). Determination of picomole amounts of dopamine, noradrenaline, DOPA, DOPAC, HVA and 5HIAA in nervous tissue after one-step purification on Sephadex G-10, using HPLC with a novel type of electrochemical detection. *J. Neurochem.* **36**, 1449–62.

Ligand Binding to Membrane Bound Neurotransmitter Receptors

6.1 Introduction

Ligand binding techniques have been successfully applied to the study of a wide range of hormone and neurotransmitter receptors, and have provided much useful information in psychopharmacology and related areas. Binding studies have been concerned not only with the properties and distribution of such receptors in the CNS, but also with the measurement of drug and hormone concentrations, the identification of putative neurotransmitters, and the generation of new information on the pathogenesis of disease states.

Neurotransmitter and hormone receptors must consist of at least two distinct functional components: first, a transmitter binding site which specifically recognises the transmitter, and secondly a 'transducer' which converts the binding of transmitter into a biochemical signal such as the synthesis of cyclic nucleotides or a change in ion permeability. Ligand binding studies are concerned only with the recognition site of receptors. It should be noted, however, that a binding site does not constitute a functional receptor; neurotransmitters and drugs possess chemically active groups which can interact non-specifically with receptor preparations and apparatus used in binding assays. Thus it is essential that a number of criteria are fulfilled in drug binding studies, and the specificity of the binding site parallels known pharmacological activity.

Historically ligand binding studies began with peripheral hormone receptors such as those for oestradiol and insulin, and the nicotinic cholinergic receptor of the electroplax of *Torpedo*. The introduction of high specific activity tritium-labelled ligands, combined with the development of rapid filtration techniques, has led to an explosion of studies. Although ligand binding assays are extremely versatile and technically very straightforward to use, it is necessary to understand the basic theoretical and methodological principles involved, and care must be taken in the interpretation of the large amounts of data which can be rapidly obtained. Many aspects of neurotransmitter receptor binding have been excellently reviewed in recent years (O'Brien, 1978; Yamamura *et al.*, 1978), and this chapter deals specifically with the use of ligand binding systems with membrane-bound receptors in psychopharmacology, with particular reference to methodological issues. No attempt will be made to discuss recent applications such as receptor solubilisation, radioreceptor assays, autoradiography of receptors and *in vivo* binding studies, which have been discussed elsewhere (see Yamamura *et al.*, 1978).

6.2 Basic receptor binding models

6.2.1 *Equilibrium binding*

The basic ligand binding model involves the reversible interaction of ligand L with a single class of receptor R, following the law of mass action:

$$R + L \underset{K_{-1}}{\overset{K_1}{\rightleftharpoons}} RL$$

where K_1 is the rate constant for association and K_{-1} the rate constant for dissociation. Thus at equilibrium:

$$\frac{[R] \cdot [L]}{[RL]} = \frac{K_{-1}}{K_1} = K_D$$

where $[R]$ = concentration of receptor, $[L]$ = concentration of ligand and $[RL]$ = concentration of receptor–ligand complex. The equation is set up according to the dissociation of receptor–ligand complex, RL, and the ratio K_{-1}/K_1 is defined as the dissociation constant, K_D. Alternatively the equilibrium binding constant K_1/K_{-1} or association constant K_A may sometimes be used.

Assuming that a finite number of receptors exist, defined as B_{MAX}, it follows that

$$[R] + [RL] = B_{MAX}$$

and hence the relationship can be derived:

$$[RL] = \frac{B_{MAX}}{1 + K_D/_L}$$

as $[RL]$ = the amount of ligand bound to receptor (B):

$$B = \frac{B_{MAX}}{1 + K_D/_L} \text{ or } B = \frac{B_{MAX}\,[L]}{K_D + [L]} \tag{6.1}$$

which is analogous to the expression of enzyme–substrate interactions, where K_D is equivalent to K_m or K_s. The K_D is frequently used as a measure of affinity of interaction between ligand and receptor and is expressed in units of concentration; the lower the value of K_D, the higher the affinity of interaction. When equation 6.1 is shown graphically, as in Fig. 6.1, it can be seen that as the ligand concentration increases the receptor population becomes increasingly occupied, with bound ligand B reaching a limiting value, B_{MAX}. When ligand concentration equals K_D, $B = \frac{1}{2} B_{MAX}$ (Eqa 6.1), i.e. 50% of the receptor population is occupied by ligand. The lower the K_D value, the lower the concentration of ligand required to occupy 50% of the receptor population. Thus in the basic receptor model the binding site population is defined by two constants, the equilibrium dissociation constant K_D and the number of binding sites B_{MAX}.

It should be noted that several assumptions are made in the derivation

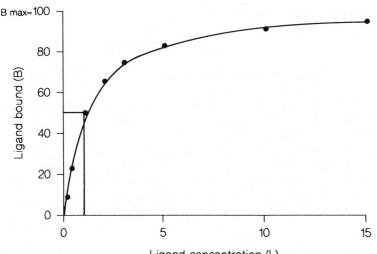

Fig. 6.1. The saturation isotherm. Data are derived from the equation $B = B_{MAX}/(1 + K_D/L)$, where maximum binding $B_{MAX} = 100$ and dissociation constant $K_D = 1$.

of simple binding isotherms. If the assumptions do not hold true, then the experimental data will deviate from the simple mass action interaction described above. These assumptions are:

(1) Binding of ligand is reversible.
(2) The receptor consists of a homogeneous, non-interacting class of binding sites, i.e. binding of one ligand molecule does not facilitate (positive co-operativity) or inhibit (negative co-operativity) the binding of subsequent ligand molecules (section 6.3).
(3) The concentration of receptor is small compared with the concentration of ligand, such that a negligible proportion of total ligand is bound.

6.2.2 *Competitive inhibition of ligand binding*
The incorporation into the simple ligand–receptor binding system of a second competing ligand I, which may be an agonist or antagonist, will result in competitive inhibition of the binding of the ligand under study,

$$R + L \underset{K_{-1}}{\overset{K_1}{\rightleftharpoons}} RL$$

$$R + I \underset{K'_{-1}}{\overset{K'_1}{\rightleftharpoons}} RI$$

The equation can be derived

$$B = \frac{B_{MAX}\,[L]}{K_D\,(1 + [I]/K_i) + (L)}$$

where $[I]$ = concentration of inhibitor, and $K_i = \dfrac{K'_{-1}}{K'_1}$ = dissociation constant of inhibitor. Thus when plotted (Fig. 6.2) a reduction in apparent affinity is evident (i.e. an increase in apparent K_D or $K_{D\ app}$) of receptor–ligand interaction with increasing inhibitor concentration, i.e. $K_{D\ app} = K_D\,(1 + ([I]/K_i))$. With increasing inhibitor concentration and a fixed ligand concentration a series of parallel displacement curves are obtained (Fig. 6.3). From these curves the concentration of inhibitor required to produce 50% inhibition of binding (IC_{50}) can be obtained and used to calculate K_i as discussed in section 6.7.2.

6.3 Methodological issues

In the investigation of membrane-bound receptors the general approach has been to study the binding of a radioactive ligand to a preparation of tissue or organelles presumed to contain the receptor, the bound ligand being separated from the unbound or free ligand by physical techniques. In most instances the number of receptors present in the preparation is extremely small, and radioactive ligands have to be of high specific activity. Moreover, the high affinity of many such binding processes (10^{-11}–10^{-9}M) necessitates the use of extremely low concentrations of ligand, again requiring high specific activity.

As the majority of receptor binding sites are present in low amounts in cellular membranes, a relatively large amount of membrane preparation is used in many ligand binding assays. The radioactive ligands used in binding studies are often lipophilic and frequently give high levels of non-specific binding (section 6.4). Whereas it has been possible to quantitatively solubilise the nicotinic receptor from muscle before labelling, this has not been possible for brain receptor binding sites and therefore means have to be found to reduce non-specific binding. Moreover, due to the presence of multiple receptor binding sites in brain and the non-selective action of many ligands, frequently ligands bind to more than one receptor site. Thus in defining specific binding great care must be taken in first excluding non-specific interactions with membranes, and secondly excluding specific interactions with other binding sites (section 6.4). Thus the specificity of the ligand binding assay and also the reliability and precision will depend not only on the choice of radioactive ligand and the agent(s) used to define specific binding, but also on the membrane preparation and technique used to separate bound from free ligand.

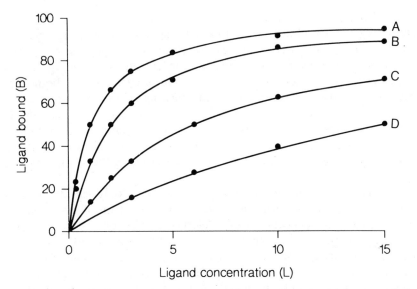

Fig. 6.2 Saturation isotherms in the presence of increasing inhibitor concentration [*I*]. Data are derived as in Fig. 6.1. for curve A [*I*] = O; B [*I*] = 1; C [*I*] = 5, and D [*I*] = 10.

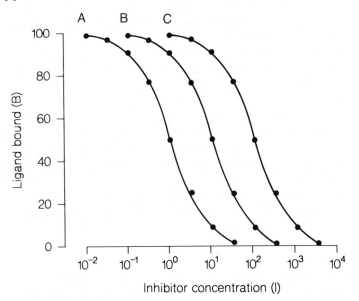

Fig. 6.3 Displacement of bound ligand by a competitive inhibitor. The inhibitor concentration is given in units of K_i, with increasing ligand concentrations. Curve A [L] = 1; B and C with increasing [L]. Bound ligand is expressed as a percentage of that bound in the absence of inhibitor.

6.3.1 *Membrane preparation*

The choice of membrane preparation to be used in binding assays is determined by a number of factors. To study the properties of receptor binding sites it may be preferable to concentrate the binding site by subcellular fractionation, e.g. by preparation of synaptic membranes. In this way less tissue is required in the binding assay, and non-specific binding may be reduced (i.e. the signal-to-noise ratio is increased). In studies requiring the comparison of receptor binding levels in a large number of different samples, it may be preferable to use a crude membrane preparation thus minimising losses and ensuring that each sample is of a similar constituency.

The choice of homogenisation procedure can only be determined empirically. Commonly used methods involve mechanical disruption in combination with sonication (e.g. Polytron PT10), or disruption alone (e.g. Ultra Turrax). These methods give reproducible homogenates, but some loss of binding may occur as compared with membranes produced with a teflon–glass homogeniser. Connective tissue is not a problem in brain tissue, and it can be removed from other tissue homogenates either by low-speed centrifugation or by filtration through muslin.

Membranes are prepared by centrifugation and are washed several times to remove substances that may interfere in the binding assay. These may be enzymes that can metabolise unbound ligand, proteins and other substances which interact non-specifically with ligand binding sites and also endogenous ligands. In some cases a straightforward homogenate can be used, for instance in muscarinic receptor binding assays where the endogenous ligand, acetylcholine, is extremely unstable and disappears rapidly after homogenisation. In other cases extensive washing is required. Thus in ^{3}H-GABA binding, membranes have to be washed at least six times and frozen-thawed to remove endogenous GABA which is present in large amounts and is very potent in ^{3}H-GABA binding assays. Details of synaptic membrane and crude total membrane preparations are given in figs 6.4 and 6.5. In many studies membranes are treated with agents to prevent metabolism of ligands, e.g. protease or monoamine oxidase inhibitors, or agents that may reduce non-specific binding, e.g. ions, detergents and albumin.

6.3.2 *Ligand*

As described earlier, because of the low numbers of binding sites and the high affinity of binding, radioactive ligands must be of high specific activity. The isotopes most commonly used are tritium and ^{125}I. Tritiated ligands are generally of the same biological activity as the parent compound, and have the advantage of a long half-life (12 years). On the other hand, though high specific activities are sometimes obtainable (i.e. >50

Tissue homogenised in 0.32 M sucrose + 50 mM tris HCl pH 7.4
↓
Centrifuge 1000 *g* 15 min
↓
Wash pellet and combine supernatants
↓
Centrifuge 9000 *g* 20 min
↓
Lyse pellet (Pz fraction) in 50 mM tris HCl pH 7.4
↓
Centrifuge 20 000 *g* 20 min
↓
Resuspend pellet in buffer for binding assay

Fig. 6.4. Preparation of crude 'synaptic' membranes.

Crude membrane preparation
↓
Tissue homogenised 40 volumes buffer 4°C
↓
Centrifuge 20 000 *g* 20 min 4°C

⊢→ discard supernatant

Resuspend pellet in original volume of buffer
↓
Centrifuge 20 000 *g* 20 min 4°C

⊢→ discard supernatant

Resuspend pellet in original volume of buffer for binding assay

Fig. 6.5. Crude membrane preparation. The scheme may differ in some details between laboratories, but in most cases a buffer of 50 mM tris HCl pH 7.4 is used.

Ci/mmol), most are in the range 10–50 Ci/mmol. In addition, the majority of laboratories have to rely on commercial preparation of ligands. For many protein and peptide hormones, iodination with ^{125}I can result in a labelled ligand of high (>200 Ci/mmol) specific activity with little loss of biological activity. The disadvantages of iodinated ligands lie in the short radiochemical half-life and chemical and radiation-induced degradation of ligand, which can, for example, reduce the biological half-life of some iodinated peptides to a few days even when stored deep-frozen.

Because of the problems involved with non-specific binding (section 6.4), radiochemical purity of ligands becomes essential. In general thin layer chromatography is the most convenient method of assessing purity of tritiated ligands, and also for repurifying ligands. Because of varying conditions of transport, packaging and storage, it is suggested that commercial preparations be checked for purity, using systems recommended by the supplier. For iodinated ligands, initial separation of ^{125}I-ligand from free iodine is sometimes followed by further purification of labelled ligand to obtain fractions with optimal binding activity. Procedures for iodination and subsequent purification have been reviewed recently (Roth, 1975).

To prevent decomposition of labelled ligands and hence to obtain reliable and reproducible results, it is essential to store ligands under optimal conditions. Commercially manufactured ligands are supplied with details of optimal storage conditions. In general, light-sensitive ligands which are readily oxidised should be stored in the dark with a suitable antioxidant. To prevent radiation-induced damage, ligands should be stored as dilute as possible in a solvent such as ethanol or methanol, which is able to remove free radicals. Storage temperatures are usually as low as possible: storage over liquid nitrogen in small aliquots to prevent freeze–thawing cycles is desirable.

6.3.3 *Incubation conditions*

To obtain reliable and reproducible results, binding assays must be performed under optimal conditions of pH, ionic strength and composition, and temperature, and with optimal concentrations of tissue preparation and ligand. These conditions are usually arrived at empirically; however, a number of general points can be made. As the amount of tissue used in assays depends ultimately on the number of receptors present, enough tissue must be used to give appreciable radioactive counts above background, i.e. 300–500 cpm. If a ligand of 10 Ci/mmol specific activity is being used, with a counting efficiency of 50% 500 cpm will correspond to 50 fmol of ligand. Assuming a receptor density of 100 fmol/mg of membrane protein and a ligand concentration equal to the K_D (i.e. 50% of receptors occupied), then 1 mg of membrane protein will be required to give 500 cpm. This assumes that non-specific binding is negligible, something which is rarely encountered. In estimating the amount of tissue to be used, linearity between amount of tissue preparation added and ligand bound has to be established. As discussed previously (section 6.2.2) (see also Rodbard, 1973), it is assumed that the amount of ligand bound is small compared with the total ligand present, such that at equilibrium total ligand approximately equals free ligand. In some cases the proportion of ligand bound may exceed 10%, in which case it is necessary to increase the incubation volume while maintaining ligand and ion concentrations but not increasing the membrane content.

In determining the length of time and temperature of incubation the most important considerations are first that equilibrium is reached (section 6.2.1) and secondly that metabolism of ligand is minimised. As the rate of association depends on ligand concentration (section 6.2.1), when a range of ligand concentrations are used, the lowest should be employed to determine the time taken to reach equilibrium. To prevent metabolism of ligands, incubations are frequently carried out at low temperatures, with subsequent increases in equilibration times. Although low-temperature incubations may prevent metabolism of ligand, it should be noted that temperature-dependent conformational changes can occur in membrane-bound proteins. Such changes are well documented for benzodiazepine receptors.

6.3.4 *Separation of bound and free ligand*

As the present discussion is restricted to membrane-bound receptors, the choice of separation technique is limited to some form of equilibrium dialysis, filtration or centrifugation. The use of equilibrium dialysis is extremely restrictive, and in general either rapid filtration or centrifugation are used. The choice between these two separation techniques depends mainly on the rate of dissociation of ligand, and to a lesser extent on the degree of non-specific binding. For rapidly dissociating ligands it is necessary to minimise separation time after equilibrium is perturbed. In many cases this is not possible even with rapid filtration techniques requiring only a few seconds of separation and wash time. This problem can be overcome by harvesting membranes by centrifugation, in which case equilibrium is not disturbed.

It should be noted that although dissociation rates can be estimated from dissociation constants by assuming a constant association rate, this is not always possible. Thus one would estimate that binding equilibria with dissociation constants of 10^{-9} M and below will have dissociation half-lives of several minutes or longer. However, for high-affinity ^{3}H-GABA binding $(K_D 10^{-9}-10^{-8}M)$ dissociation is too rapid to allow estimates even at 4°C.

The most commonly used separation technique for membrane-bound receptors would seem to be rapid filtration. Once incubations have reached equilibrium, they are rapidly diluted with cold buffer and passed over the filter, followed by several washes with cold buffer. The time taken for such a procedure is generally less than 20 s. A variety of apparatus is available from commercial sources, varying from a single support for one 2.5 cm filter to large manifolds supporting 30 or more filters in banks designed to give equal filtration rates under reduced pressure. The choice of filters is again empirical, those used most commonly being glass-fibre filters of the Whatman GF B/C type. Whatever type of filter is used, the binding of ligand to filters in the absence of tissue should be minimised thus reducing non-specific interactions (section 6.4). More recently a semi-automated technique has been developed based on the use of cell-harvesting equipment. Such systems are useful for the processing of samples from a large number of assays, and are described in detail elsewhere (Hall and Thor, 1979).

Although centrifugation has to be used in some cases where dissociation of the ligand is extremely rapid, in general non-specific binding of ligands is greater due to the less efficient washing of the tissue. In this instance, non-specific binding is composed of that amount bound to the tissue and a further amount trapped in the pellet. Care must be taken to wash the centrifuge tube and surface of the pellet to remove as much extraneous ligand as possible. By using high-speed microcentrifuges, large numbers of samples can be rapidly and conveniently processed.

Detailed protocols for the binding of ligands to dopamine receptors are given in the next section.

6.4 Practical example: ligand binding to dopamine receptors

The binding of neuroleptic drugs to dopamine receptors may be associated with at least two types of dopamine receptor (Kebabian and Calne, 1979). In this example, ^{3}H-spiperone is used as a ligand for one class of dopamine receptor, the D2 receptor, and ^{3}H-piflutixol as ligand for the D1 receptor (Hyttel, 1982).

6.4.1 *Membrane preparation*

Highest levels of dopamine receptors are found in striatum (caudate putamen) and hence this is used as the tissue source. The same crude membrane preparation may be used for both ligand binding assays.

(1) Rat striata (100 mg tissue) homogenised in 40 volumes (4 ml) of 50 mM tris/HCl buffer, pH 7.4 at 4°C, using an Ultra Turrax (or Polytron PT-10) for 10 s.

(2) Centrifuge homogenate 20 000 g for 20 min at 4°C.

(3) Discard supernatant, rehomogenise pellet in 4.0 ml 50 mM tris HCl Ph 7.4.

(4) Recentrifuge, 20 000 g for 20 min at 4°C.

(5) Discard supernatant, rehomogenise pellet in 4.0 ml 50 mM tris HCl pH 7.4 and keep on ice for binding assay. The membrane preparation may be stored at −40°C with slight loss of binding activity. Alternatively the pellet may be stored at −40°C after the final centrifugation and reconstituted for the binding assay with minimal

loss of binding activity. Storage of membrane preparations at 4°C for long periods (i.e. greater than 2 h) may result in substantial losses of binding activity.

6.4.2 *^{3}H-Spiperone binding*
Assay tubes are set up in triplicate containing ^{3}H-spiperone 25–30 Ci/mmol) and the following:

For total binding:	*For non-specific binding:*
200 μl membrane preparation	200 μl membrane preparation
100 μl ^{3}H-spiperone (5 nM)	100 μl ^{3}H-spiperone (5 nM)
600 μl 50 mM tris HCl pH 7.4	600 μl 50 mM tris HCl pH 7.4
100 μl 1 μM (−)butaclamol	100 μl 1 μM (+)butaclamol

$$\downarrow$$
Incubate 37°C 20 min
$$\downarrow$$

To each tube is added 5 ml ice-cold 50 mM tris HCl pH 7.4, the contents are passed over 2.5 cm Whatman GFB filter, and each tube is washed out over the filter twice with 5 ml aliquots of ice-cold buffer.

$$\downarrow$$

Filters mixed with water-miscible scintillant and allowed to equilibrate 6 h before counting.

6.4.3 *^{3}H-Piflutixol binding*
Assay tubes are set up containing:

Total binding:	*Non-specific binding:*
800 μl membrane preparation	800 μl membrane preparation
100 μl ^{3}H-piflutixol (5 nM)	100 μl ^{3}H-piflutixol (5 nM)
1100 μl 50 mM tris HCl pH 7.4	1000 μl tris HCl pH 7.4
	100 μl 20 μM (+)butaclamol

$$\downarrow$$
Incubate 37°C for 20 min
$$\downarrow$$

Tubes filtered as for ^{3}H-spiperone binding, except that Whatman GFC filters and four washes of buffer are used.

Some points about the differences in these binding assays are:

(1) A larger incubation volume is used for ^{3}H-piflutixol as proportionally more of the ligand is bound than ^{3}H-spiperone. Under these conditions less than 10% of total ligand is bound for both assays (see section 6.3.3).

(2) The different filtration methods are used to minimise ^{3}H-piflutixol

binding to the glass-fibre filters. Using Whatman GFB glass fibre filters and only three buffer washes for ^{3}H-piflutixol results in high levels of filter binding, some of which may be displaced by unlabelled neuroleptics (see section 6.4).

(3) The greater amount of tissue used in section 6.4.3 is due to the low specific activity of ^{3}H-piflutixol.

(4) For spiperone binding, specific binding is defined as the difference in ligand bound in the presence of (+) and (−) isomers of butaclamol, for ^{3}H-piflutixol specific binding is that displaced by (+)butaclamol (section 6.4).

6.5 Non-specific binding

As mentioned earlier, and described in detail elsewhere (Hollenberg and Cuatrecasas, 1978), binding of radioactive ligands even at low concentrations ($<10^{-9}$ M) will involve interactions not only with the receptor under study but also with many other structures. A large proportion of the drugs used as ligands are by design highly lipid-soluble and contain many reactive groups, and thus their capacity for high non-specific binding is not surprising. The distinction between specific and non-specific binding is dependent on the specificity and potency of the ligand used, the choice of tissue source and the operational criteria adopted to define specific binding.

In most cases the nature of the components involved in non-specific binding is unknown. However, one can envisage several different types of non-specific binding which will depend to a certain extent on the nature of the study undertaken. Thus if ligand binding is used to investigate the mode of action of a particular drug, non-specific binding may be defined as that not involving a high-affinity receptor, i.e. simply ligand dissolved in the lipid phase of membranes, associated with membrane-bound ions and proteins, etc. In this case non-specific binding would be of high capacity and low affinity, and specific binding may involve several membrane components all of which may be relevant to the mode of action of the drug used as ligand. On the other hand, if one is using a ligand purely as a probe to study a defined binding site, then the criteria for specific binding become more stringent. In this case specific binding will involve only the high-affinity site under question, and non-specific binding may include other high-affinity binding sites along with high-capacity low-affinity sites. These distinctions become more relevant in the case of a ligand that interacts with more than one transmitter receptor site, a situation often encountered.

There are basically two techniques available for the determination of specific and non-specific binding. By measuring binding over a wide range of concentrations and by subsequent analysis of the data (section 6.7) one can demonstrate the presence of multiple saturable components and also non-saturable (i.e. truly non-specific) binding. A more commonly used procedure involves displacement of ligand from binding sites by the inclusion of competing drugs in the incubation. From the description of competitive inhibition given in section 6.7.3 it can be calculated that when the ligand concentration is equal to K_D then a $100 \times K_i$ concentration of inhibitor will give practically total displacement of ligand. The choice of displacing drug once again depends on the type of study undertaken. Thus to displace ligand from all high-affinity sites an excess of unlabelled ligand or a structurally closely related drug can be used. In this case non-specific binding will consist of low-affinity high-capacity interactions. To study the binding of ligand to a pharmacologically well-defined receptor, it is preferable to use a displacing agent of the required specificity which is structurally unrelated to the ligand. In this case non-specific binding may consist of high-affinity binding to other receptors as well as low-affinity binding.

An example of these considerations is given by the binding of the ligand ^{3}H-spiperone, initially proposed as a ligand for dopamine receptors in brain (Fields *et al.*, 1977). When unlabelled spiperone is used, a large proportion of the binding is displaced (Fig. 6.6). However, if the specific dopamine antagonist sulpiride (which is structurally unrelated to spiperone) is used, considerably less of the binding is displaced, suggesting that several high-affinity binding sites may be present. Subsequent analysis with the serotonin antagonist ketanserin and butaclamol (which binds to serotonin and dopamine receptors) suggests that ^{3}H-spiperone may bind with high affinity not only to dopamine receptors, but also to serotonin receptors and to a site specific for some part of the spiperone molecule (Fig. 6.6). By using spiperone to define non-specific binding, three high-affinity 'specific' binding sites can be delineated, all of which may contribute to the pharmacological activity of spiperone. In using ^{3}H-spiperone as a ligand for dopamine receptors, the contribution of these other high-affinity binding sites must be prevented by using a specific dopamine antagonist unrelated in structure to spiperone, e.g. sulpiride.

In defining non-specific binding the criterion of stereoselectivity has proved extremely useful. In many pharmacological systems activity is found to reside in one stereoisomer of an optically active drug. Thus in binding assays at an appropriate concentration the active isomer will displace labelled ligand from the binding site whereas the inactive isomer will not. It is assumed that non-specific displacement of ligand will be equivalent for both isomers. Although stereospecific displacement is useful in defining purely non-specific binding, a number of problems have

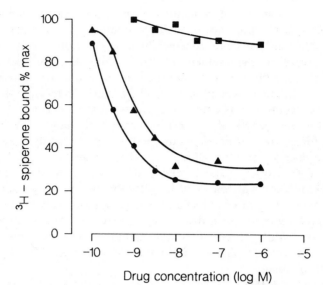

Fig. 6.6. Interactions of spiperone (●), (+)butaclamol (▲), and ketanserin (■) with ^{3}H-spiperone binding in calf caudate membranes. The ^{3}H-spiperone displaced by 10^{-6} M ketanserin represents binding to serotonin receptors; that displaced by 10^{-6} M (+)butaclamol includes both serotonin and dopamine receptors. The difference between (+)butaclamol and spiperone represents binding to the 'spirodecanone site'.

been encountered. Therefore in defining the binding of ligands to dopamine receptors, the optical isomers of the neuroleptic butaclamol are frequently used (section 6.4.3), (+)butaclamol being active and (−)butaclamol inactive at dopamine receptors (Fig. 6.7). It has become clear, however, that the butaclamol isomers are also differentially active at serotonin receptors, leading to possible artefacts.

The factors discussed above clearly demonstrate the need to reduce non-specific binding as far as possible. When non-specific binding includes high-affinity saturable sites, these can be blocked by the addition of appropriate inhibitors. In the case of ^{3}H-spiperone binding to dopamine receptors, non-specific binding (which includes serotonin and spirodecanone components) can be reduced by the addition of a serotonin antagonist and spirodecanone, both of which are inactive at dopamine receptors. Low-affinity non-specific binding can be reduced in some instances by the addition of anti-absorbents such as serum albumin in the case of peptide ligands. In some cases such binding can be reduced by modulation of ionic strength and composition, and pH. In all cases the efficiency of the washing procedure should be determined experimentally.

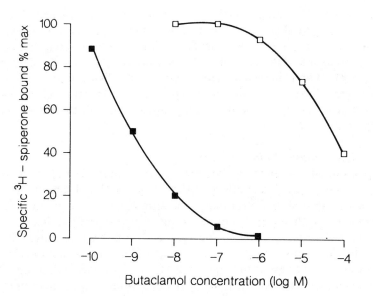

Fig. 6.7. Stereospecific displacement of ³H-spiperone binding to calf caudate membranes by (+)butaclamol (□) and (−)butaclamol (■).

6.6 Criteria for receptor specific binding

6.6.1 *Saturability*

From the basic model of receptor binding interactions (section 6.2) a number of criteria for the definition of receptor specific binding are evident. First, a finite number of binding sites are present, and thus with increasing concentrations of ligand the proportion of binding sites occupied will increase until all are occupied (i.e. saturation). For most ligands the number of binding sites in brain varies from 50 to 500 fmol/mg of membrane protein, but this is not always the case. Some peptide binding sites may be present at levels of 5 fmol/mg protein, and amino acid binding sites may be present at several picomoles per miligram of protein. In most cases the affinity of the ligand determined from saturation experiments should be consistent with its biological effects. Saturability of ligand binding can also be demonstrated as a competitive inhibition of binding by the addition of increasing concentrations of unlabelled ligand.

A second criterion arising from the basic model is that of reversibility (section 6.2.1). Thus if binding is allowed to reach equilibrium and then free ligand is effectively removed from the incubation, there will be a progressive decrease in the amount of ligand bound until a new equilibrium is reached. Experimentally the removal of free ligand from the incubation can be achieved either by a large dilution of the incubation mixture, or by the addition of a large excess of unlabelled ligand or other displacing agent (Fig. 6.8). From these experiments the rate constant of dissociation (K_{-1}) can be calculated, and similarly from time-course experiments the rate constant of association (K_1) can be determined (Fig. 6.8). When these data are obtained, the dissociation constant can be calculated from the relationship $K_D = K_{-1}/K_1$ (Section 6.2.1). The K_D calculated as above should be in good agreement with the value obtained from equilibrium binding.

6.6.2 *Distribution of binding sites*
In general, specific binding sites for a ligand should be present in tissues where a pharmacological effect of the ligand can be observed. Although the distribution of neurotransmitter or drug receptors need not necessarily correlate with the distribution of the neurotransmitter itself, for the binding site to be relevant to the actions of a given transmitter, binding sites should be present in responsive tissues. This applies not only to gross distribution in organs of the body, but also to distribution in distinct brain regions and subcellular fractions. Thus one would expect neurotransmitter receptor binding sites to be concentrated in synaptic membranes.

6.6.3 *Comparative potencies of drugs*
The basis of identification of a given receptor depends primarily on its pharmacology. Thus a comparison can be made between the efficacies of a range of drugs in inhibiting ligand binding and in producing a physiological effect. The identification of a ligand binding site as a pharmacologically relevant receptor can be made on the basis of the comparative potency of a range of drugs. As discussed earlier, the IC_{50} or K_i value can be taken as a measure of potency in ligand binding systems. These values can be compared with similar measures of potency (e.g. ED_{50}) obtained from dose–response experiments in biological assays. In many instances the affinities of drugs in ligand binding assays may not be directly comparable with their affinities estimated from dose–response curves. This is particularly true in the case of agonists, where the physiological response is several steps removed from the binding of agonist to receptor. More directly comparable information can be obtained from the action of antagonists. The models of antagonist competitively blocking the action of agonist are independent of the relationship between agonist interaction with receptor and subsequent biological response. The equations derived from these models are analogous to those used in binding studies, and form the basis of simple receptor binding models (section 6.2).

A comparison of the relative potencies of a range of antagonists in ligand binding with their biological activity provides a powerful tool in receptor identification. An example of this is given by the potency of

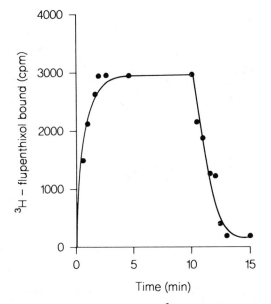

Fig. 6.8. Association and dissociation of ^{3}H-flupenthixol 1.0 nM with calf caudate membranes. To determine dissociation, 500 nM unlabelled flupenthixol was added at $t = 10$ min.

neuroleptic drugs in inhibiting ^{3}H-spiperone binding to dopamine receptors and their clinical efficacy (Fig. 6.9). It is also important in this type of study to show that structurally related drugs which are pharmacologically inactive are also inactive in the ligand binding assay, and that drugs active at other receptors are similarly inactive.

6.7 Analysis of binding data

6.7.1 *Saturation data*

As outlined in section 6.2, the determination of maximum binding capacity (B_{MAX}) and dissociation constant (K_D) from equilibrium binding involves incubating a fixed amount of receptor with increasing concentrations of ligand. The resulting saturation curve (Fig. 6.1) in the case of a single class of binding sites should conform to a rectangular hyperbola. As in enzyme kinetics, a number of linear transformations of these data are possible, and in general two transformations are frequently encountered. The basic receptor interaction described by

$$B = \frac{B_{MAX} [L]}{K_D + [L]}$$

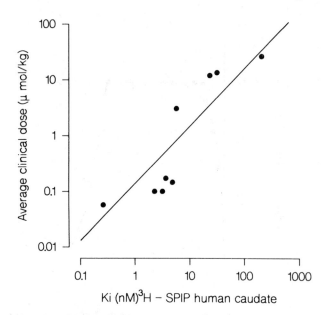

Fig. 6.9. Relationship of clinical potency of neuroleptics to potency in ^{3}H-spiperone binding to human caudate membranes.

can be transformed to the Scatchard equation (Scatchard, 1949):

$$B/[L] = \frac{B_{MAX}}{K_D} - \frac{B}{K_D}$$

or to the Klotz (Klotz and Huntson, 1971) equation, which is equivalent to the double reciprocal plot:

$$\frac{1}{B} = \frac{K_D}{B_{MAX}} \cdot \frac{1}{[L]} \frac{1}{B_{MAX}}$$

An example of the Scatchard linear transformation and the derivation of constants is given in Fig. 6.10. For the graphical determination of K_D and B_{MAX}, extrapolation of lines to the axes must be made. This may be difficult in both cases: as B/F or $1/F$ approach zero $[L]$ becomes large, and as $[L]$ increases, non-specific binding increases, thus increasing the error in the determination of ligand bound, B. The double reciprocal plot also suffers from the fact that an inverse function of $[L]$ is being used, which results in compression of the range as $[L]$ increases. In general the Scatchard plot is preferred to the double reciprocal plot, if only because of the more even distribution of the points (see, for example, Klotz and Huntson, 1971). If lines are fitted by linear regression analysis, both transformations yield identical results. However, in double reciprocal

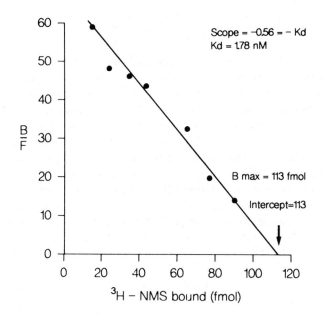

Fig. 6.10. Saturation analysis and Scatchard plot. Data are presented for the binding of ^{3}H–N methyl scopolamine to rat cortical muscarinic receptors. Non-specific binding was determined using 1 μM atropine. The data were derived from the following experiment:

Ligand added (cpm)	Ligand (nM)	Total binding (cpm)	Non-specific binding (cpm)	Specific binding (cpm)	Bound ^{3}H-NMS (fmol)	Bound/free (fmol/nM)
6 873	0.25	711	33	678	14.7	59.0
13 725	0.30	1 138	39	1 101	23.9	47.8
20 745	0.75	1 654	49	1 605	34.9	46.5
27 657	1.0	2 065	58	2 007	43.6	43.6
55 017	2.0	3 091	84	3 007	65.3	32.7
111 777	4.1	3 670	147	3 522	76.5	18.7
164 985	6.0	4 099	205	3 894	84.7	14.1

plots more weighting may be given by eye to those points derived from the lowest values of B and $[L]$, which may be the least accurate.

6.7.2 Inhibition data

To determine K_i values of inhibitors, a fixed concentration of receptor preparation and binding ligand are present, and increasing concentrations of competing drug are used. In the presence of competing drug, ligand binding is described by the equation:

$$B = \frac{B_{MAX}\,[L]}{K_D\,(1 + [I]/K_i) + [L]}$$

Thus as the concentration of competing drug increases, the amount of ligand progressively decreases to give the typical dose–response curve shown in Fig. 6 .11. Due to the nature of the curve, the determination of IC_{50} values directly is inaccurate. A number of linear transformations of the data are available to facilitate the determination of IC_{50} values from inhibition curves. A frequently encountered technique is that of probit analysis. In this case the amount of ligand bound is expressed as fractional occupancy, and these values can be converted to probit values using the appropriate statistical tables. By plotting these probit values against log $[I]$ a linear relationship is obtained and IC_{50} values can be calculated from linear regression analysis (Fig. 6.11). The equilibrium dissociation constant of the inhibitor (K_i) can be calculated from the equation (Cheng and Prusoff, 1973):

$$K_i = \frac{IC_{50}}{1 + [L]/K_D}$$

It should be noted that as the concentration of ligand decreases to values well below the K_D the IC_{50} value approaches the K_i. If unlabelled ligand is used as displacing agent, then the K_i value is equivalent to the K_D. This provides a simple method for the approximate estimation of K_D for a ligand of unknown affinity.

6.7.3 *Hill plots*
A further linear transformation of inhibition or saturation data is the Hill plot. This analysis has the advantage of providing additional information on the mode of interaction between receptor and ligand. Hill plots occupy a central position in ligand binding studies where there is more than one apparent number of binding sites. If n is the number of apparent binding sites on a receptor, then the reaction can be described by:

$$R + nL \rightleftharpoons RL_n$$

the binding isotherm is then described by

$$B = \frac{B_{MAX}\,[L]n}{K'_D + [L]n}$$

which is the Hill equation, and may be transformed to

$$\log \frac{B}{(B_{MAX} - B)} = n \log [L] - \log K'_D$$

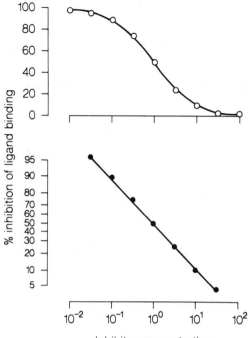

Fig. 6.11.   Inhibition of ligand binding by competitive inhibitor. Upper: ligand binding as a function of inhibitor concentration. Lower: log-probit plot of the inhibition data. Data as in Fig. 6.3, inhibition concentration in units of IC$_{50}$.

In this case K'_D is the apparent dissociation constant. When log $B/(B_{MAX} - B)$ is plotted against log L, the slope of the line equals the apparent stoichiometry of the interaction. Both saturation and inhibition data can be fitted to the equation. For inhibition data the fractional occupancy function is used:

$$\log [\%I/(100 - \%I)] = n \log [I] - \log IC_{50}$$

Examples of saturation and inhibition data fitted to these equations are shown in Fig. 6.12.

A number of qualitative conclusions can be derived from Hill plots. The Hill constant, n (or n_H) is equal to 1 when only one class of non-interacting binding sites is present. If the Hill coefficient is less than one, this suggests that either negative co-operativity is present or more than one class of binding site is involved. Negative co-operativity will be apparent when the binding of one ligand molecule reduces the affinity of subsequent ligand–receptor interactions. It follows that ligand binding sites are not independent, i.e. they are linked via some allosteric interac-

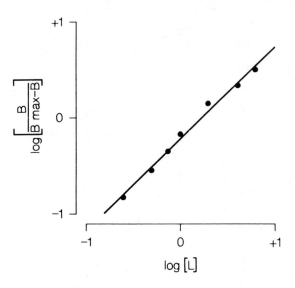

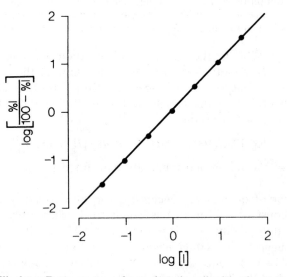

Fig. 6.12. Hill plots. Data are transformed as described in the text. Upper: for saturation analysis, data from Fig. 6.1. Lower: for inhibition studies, data from Fig. 6.3.

tion (Monod *et al.*, 1965). The Hill coefficient will be greater than unity in the case of positive co-operativity. It should be noted that n_H is dependent upon $[L]$ and therefore if the slope of the line is less than one for a given $[L]$, it is possible that there may be more than one class of binding site involved in the interaction at that ligand concentration. At either extreme of saturation n_H will always equal unity as ligand is interacting initially at low concentration only with the highest affinity site, while at high concentration the low-affinity site is saturated and it is interacting only with the lowest affinity site (Fig. 6.13). It follows that classes of site are determined solely by their affinity for ligand; physically distinct sites with equal affinity for ligand will not be distinguished by this analysis.

6.8 Receptor heterogeneity

6.8.1 *Multiple binding sites and allosteric interactions*
It has become increasingly evident in recent years that just as enzymes may exist in several distinct molecular forms, so too may drug and neurotransmitter receptors. Instances of receptor heterogeneity have been identified by classical pharmacology and have been known for many years. Included in this group are muscarinic and nicotinic cholinergic receptors, α- and β-adrenergic receptors, and histamine H_1 and H_2 receptors. Ligand binding techniques have verified receptor heterogeneity in

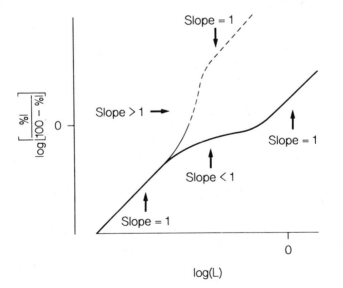

Fig. 6.13. Non-linear Hill plots. At the limits of ligand concentration $[L]$, slope = 1, slope may deviate from unity at intermediate concentrations. Solid line, negative co-operativity; dashed line, positive co-operativity.

these examples, and also a great deal of evidence has accumulated from similar studies indicating the presence of receptor heterogeneity in many other pharmacological systems.

As discussed in the previous section, receptor heterogeneity can only be detected in equilibrium binding systems on the basis of different dissociation constants or K_D values. Thus for two receptors of dissociation constants K_1 and K_2, the binding isotherm is described by:

$$B = \frac{B_{\text{MAX}_1} [L]}{K_1 + [L]} + \frac{B_{\text{MAX}_2} [L]}{K_2 + [L]}$$

When saturation data from this two-site model are plotted by the method of Scatchard, a curve is produced which is the sum of the two independent binding functions (Fig. 6.14). The asymptotes of the curve represent binding to the individual sites, the shape of the curve depending on the relative affinities of the sites. In the case of Hill plots a non-linear relationship is produced as described in the previous section (Fig. 6.13).

The presence of non-linear Scatchard and Hill plots does not prove the existence of multiple binding sites. Although consistent with the presence of multiple sites, non-linear plots can also result from several possible

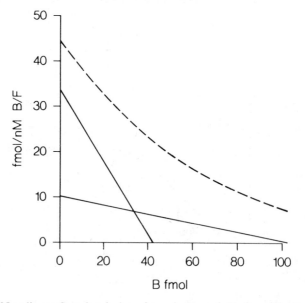

Fig. 6.14. Non-linear Scatchard plot of two independent sites. The curve results from the sum of contributions from two independent sites differing in affinity for ligand.

artefacts and also from receptor co-operativity and allosteric interactions (e.g. Chang *et al.*, 1975; Hollenberg and Cuatrecasas, 1978). It is not possible to distinguish between multiple binding sites and allosteric interactions at a single site in simple equilibrium binding experiments. Among the most common artefacts producing non-linear Scatchard plots are first the presence of non-specific interactions and secondly the use of high receptor : ligand ratios. If the complete binding isotherm of ligand, including non-specific binding, is included in a Scatchard plot, the result will be a curve (Fig. 6.15). One limit will describe saturable binding, and the other describes non-specific non-saturable binding, and reaches a limiting value of $B/[F]$ at infinite ligand bound (Chamness and McGuire, 1975). If each free concentration of ligand is multiplied by this factor, an estimate of the non-specific binding can be made. When corrected for this factor a linear relationship is obtained (Fig. 6.15). A similar plot is produced if non-specific binding has been incorrectly determined in binding experiments, e.g. by using a large excess of unlabelled ligand which results in some non-specific displacement of labelled ligand.

It has been stressed throughout that for binding experiments at equilibrium, less than 10% of total ligand should be bound, so that total ligand

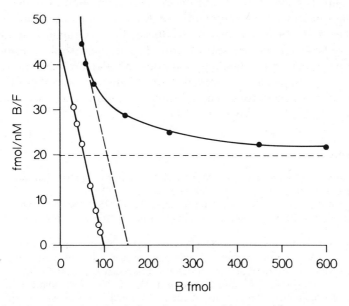

Fig. 6.15. Non-linear Scatchard plot of one saturable site and one non-saturable site. Open circles represent binding to the saturable site only, after subtraction of the non-saturable site.

approximates to free ligand concentration. If more than 10% of total ligand is bound, calculation of free ligand concentration can be made by subtraction of total bound from total ligand present. This correction cannot be made in the determination of IC_{50} values, however, and in this case it has been shown that IC_{50} values will increase as a function of receptor concentration and can in extreme cases lead to non-linear Hill plots (Chang *et al.*, 1975).

In some cases two distinct binding sites may be present which have equal affinity for the binding ligand but differing affinities for displacing agents. In this case Scatchard and Hill analyses of saturation binding data will be consistent with only one binding site. Displacement of ligand by the site-selective agent will result in flattened displacement curves which are clearly biphasic when affinities differ by 1000-fold.

6.8.2 *Calculation of apparent binding parameters for a two-site model*

A number of techniques are available for the calculation of binding parameters from saturation isotherms. When data for two-site binding are presented as a Scatchard plot, the resulting curve (Fig. 6.15) can be analysed graphically to yield two component lines (e.g. Rosenthal, 1967). These methods suffer from the problems of curve-fitting by eye and the extra weighting given to the least accurate points. A more satisfactory procedure is computerised non-linear regression analysis of the original binding isotherm. These problems are discussed in more detail elsewhere (Vallner *et al.*, 1976; Thakur and Rodbard, 1979). Graphical methods are also available for the analysis of drug displacement studies, using linear transformations of the binding isotherms. Similar problems are encountered in the graphical determination of parameters from these data, and once again computerised curve-fitting procedures are preferred (see Chapter 7, 7.3.2 and Appendix 7.1).

References

Chamness, G.C. and McGuire, W.L. (1975). Scatchard plots: common errors in correction and interpretation. *Steroids,* **26**, 538–42.

Chang, K-J., Jacobs, S. and Cuatrecasas, P. (1975). Quantitative aspects of hormone-receptor interactions of high affinity. *Biochem. Biophys. Acta* **406**, 294–303.

Cheng, Y-C. and Prusoff, W.H. (1973). Relationship between the inhibition constant (K_1) and the concentration of inhibitor which causes 50 percent inhibition of an enzymatic reaction. *Biochem. Pharmacol.* **22**, 3099–108.

Fields, J.Z., Reisine, T.D. and Yamamura, H.I. (1977). Biochemical demonstration of dopaminergic receptors in rat and human brain using ^{3}H-spiroperidol. *Brain Res.* **136**, 578–84.

Hall, H. and Thor, L. (1979) Evaluation of a semi-automatic filtration technique for receptor binding studies. *Life Sci.* **24**, 2293–300.

Hollenberg, M. and Cuatrecasas, P. (1978) Distinction of receptor from non-receptor interactions in binding studies. In *The Receptors: a Comprehensive Treatise* (R.D. O'Brien, Ed.), Plenum Press, New York.

Hyttel, J. (1981) Similarities between the binding of ^{3}H-piflutixol and ^{3}H-flupenthixol to rat striatal dopamine receptors *in vitro*. *Life Sci.* **28**, 563–8.

Kebabian, J.W. and Calne, D.B. (1979) Multiple receptors for dopamine. *Nature* **277**, 93–5.

Klotz, I.M. and Huntson, D.L. (1971) Properties of graphical representations of multiple classes of binding sites. *Biochemistry* **10**, 3065–9.

Monod, J., Wyman, J. and Changeaux, J-P. (1965) On the nature of allosteric transitions: a plausible model. *J. Mol. Biol.* **12**, 88–118.

O'Brien, R.D. (ed.) (1978) *The Receptors: a Comprehensive Treatise*, Plenum Press, New York.

Rodbard, D. (1973) Mathematics of hormone-receptor interactions. In *Receptors for Reproductive Hormones* (B.W. O'Malley and A.R. Means Eds), 289–342, Plenum Press, New York.

Rosenthal, H.E. (1967) A graphic method for the determination and presentation of binding parameters in a complex system. *Anal. Biochem.* **20**, 525–32.

Roth, J. (1975) Methods for assessing immunologic and biologic properties of iodinated peptide hormones. In *Methods in Enzymology, XXXVI*, (B.W. O'Malley and J.G. Mackman, Eds), 223–32, Academic Press, New York.

Scatchard, G. (1949) The attractions of proteins for small molecules and ions. *Ann. NY Acad. Sci.* **51**, 660–72.

Thakur, A.K. and Rodbard, D. (1979) Graphical aids to interpretation of Scatchard plots and dose–response curves. *J. Theor. Biol.* **80**, 383–403.

Vallner, J.J., Perrin, J.H. and Wold, S. (1976) Comparison of graphical cell computerised methods for calculating binding parameters for two strongly bound drugs to human serum albumin. *J. Pharm. Sci.* **65**, 1182–7.

Yamamura, H.I., Enna, S.T. and Kumar, M.J. (eds) (1978) *Neurotransmitter Receptor Binding*, Raven Press, New York.

Appendix 6.1   Trouble shooting

Problem	Possible source	Detection
1. No detectable specific binding	Ligand purity	Analysis of radiochemical purity, i.e. TLC, HPLC
	Ligand stability during incubation	Analysis of ligand metabolite HPLC, TLC
	Separation time too slow	Analyse parallel incubations by filtration and centrifugation
	Incubation conditions	Time course, temperature dependence and ionic requirements for binding
	Incorrect displacing agent	Use unlabelled ligand to displace
	Tissue source	Tissue unstable during either preparation or incubation
2. Non-saturable binding	Non-specific displacement from tissue	Assess non-specific binding with different agents
	Ligand binding to filters, tubes, etc.	Check free ligand concentration during incubation
	Equilibrium not reached at low ligand concentration	Time course of association at lowest ligand concentration
3. Incorrect dissociation constant	Ligand metabolism	Section 6.1
	Receptor concentration too high	Greater than 10% of free ligand bound
	Ligand purity and metabolism	Section 6.1
	Incubation conditions	Section 6.1

7 *Christopher D. Frith, Stephen J. Gamble and Michael H. Joseph*

Data collection and analysis

7.1 Introduction

In any experiment, as the number of variables being measured on the same set of subjects increases, storage and analysis of results become more of a practical problem. With the development of multidimensional behavioural assessment, of more sensitive analytical methods, and of methods for analysing several chemical species concurrently, problems of data handling increase in animal experiments also. In human studies, lack of experimental control over many relevant variables has always necessitated detailed analysis of results in relation to differences between subjects. The scarcity of certain clinical material, e.g. from drug-free psychiatric patients, will reinforce the tendency to make multiple observations on each subject, and give rise to other relevant variables: length of illness, previous treatments, clinical subtype, clinical course, etc.

Computers are increasingly available for the storage and analysis of experimental results. It may be argued that the corresponding increase in the availability of calculators and microcomputers will provide the necessary statistical facilities, but it is our experience that data storage and analysis by computer, usually mainframe (a large central installation shared by many users) has definite advantages. Once assembled, data can be accessed indefinitely and readily updated, especially with interactive systems. Different combinations of data can be examined and printed for use by different individuals. The biggest advantage, however, is that statistical tests and plots of the data can be obtained directly. In our opinion the risks of over-analysis of the data, and selective reporting of significant results, are outweighed by the risks that correlations, or group differences, say, will not be checked because of the need to enter the results manually.

The next two sections of this chapter will therefore briefly discuss the advantages of using (usually micro-) computers in process control and data acquisition and the advantages of using (usually mainframe) computers in data storage and data processing. The final section deals with the selection of statistical procedures and tests for the analysis of data collected. We intend that the information given here will be of direct use to the more experienced reader, but it is hoped that it will also give the less experienced a basis for discussing their requirements with specialists in these fields.

Data processing can be defined as 'the operations performed on data, usually by automatic equipment, in order to derive information or to achieve order in files' (Chandor, 1979). It should be understood that data processing therefore includes the manual manipulation of data and is not only a function of automated equipment (the computer). This point is illustrated in section 7.4.3, where various pre-analysis data cleansing operations are discussed. In the space available here, only a general introduction to data processing can be given. For more detailed information, an introductory text on data processing such as Anderson (1979) or Woolbridge (1976) should be consulted. Medical computing is dealt with specifically by Siemasko (1978) and in the guide from the Association of Clinical Biochemists (1983). The growing use of computers has led to many journals devoting special issues to the subject, e.g. *Nucleic Acids Research* (1984) and *Medical Laboratory Sciences* (1980). The *British Medical Journal* (1983) has also published a weekly series ('ABC of Computing') introducing various aspects of the use of computers in medicine.

The computer can also be used to maximum advantage where large and repetitive tasks are to be carried out, or where a number of operations need to be performed at accurately (or closely) timed intervals. It would be pointless investing large amounts of time and money acquiring a computer to do a once and for all calculation. Besides the computer, the additional cost of purchasing or writing suitable programs to run on the computer is often overlooked. The software, as sets of program instructions are called, may cost as much as a suitable computer — say £600 to £700 for a Commodore PET or an Apple II. A program is just the instructions which need to be carried out to perform a given task, and as such it is just like any other laboratory method. In a chemical method you might be required to find one tube, label it 'A', then find a second tube, label this 'B', then add the contents of tube 'A' to the contents of tube 'B' and make a note of the new volume of solution in tube 'B'. A computer might use a similar solution to add two numbers together, for example:

```
10 READ A              ! FIND THE FIRST NUMBER
20 READ B              ! FIND THE SECOND NUMBER
30 LET TOTAL = A + B   ! Add the two numbers together then
                       ! remember this answer is the total
```

The computer carries out each step of the program in the sequence given by the numbers at the beginning of each line. Text following the ! are comments to assist the user, and do not form part of the instruction.

These instructions are written in a computer language called BASIC, which stands for Beginners All-purpose Symbolic Instruction Code. The computer will then use an interpreter to translate instructions written in BASIC into its machine code, and carry them out in sequence. Other widely used computer languages are FORTRAN (FORmula TRANslation), COBOL (COmmon Business Oriented Language) and Pascal, although there are many more. Each computer language has its own advantages and disadvantages. For example FORTRAN is good for evaluating complex mathematical formulae, but not very good for use with text strings, whereas COBOL is excellent for keeping check of laboratory inventories but has limited mathematical ability. The reader who would like to find out more about given languages is recommended to consult texts such as Alcock (1977) and Munro (1974) for BASIC, Munro (1975) or Alcock (1982) for FORTRAN and Parkin (1975) for COBOL.

As with any other laboratory method, developing a computer method to solve a problem can take a lot of time. Computers are very useful where the same task needs to be performed many times. This is really the first stage of systems analysis: do we really need to use a computer or is there some other, better way to achieve the desired result? Most of the commercially available programs are designed for doing these repetitive tasks such as laboratory integration (mathematical processing of the output from instruments, e.g. Gilson Data Master System) and statistics. We have used quite extensively the statistical packages BMDP (Department of Biomathematics, University of California, Los Angeles), Minitab (Statistics Department, University of Pennsylvania) and SPP (Supersoft, Harrow, Middlesex) for analysis of data. These are available for a wide range of computers. For example, SPP, which was originally available for the Commodore PET, can now be used on Commodore 64, Sirius 1, Apple II. Apricot, IBM and other personal computers. This means that you may be able to use a version of the statistics package with which you are familiar, even if the available computing facilities change.

7.2 Process control and data collection

7.2.1 *Control of psychological test apparatus*
The speed of the computer is ideal for process control. This speed allows it to monitor switch closures, interpret them, and alter its response accordingly. The response could be lighting different lamps, sounding buzzers or closing relays. This is employed, for instance, in the control of a Skinner box used in learning tasks. If the test subject presses the correct lever, the computer detects the correct response and gives a reward; the machine then presents the next stimulus as determined by its pre-programmed strategy. It is possible for the machine to alter strategy once

the subject reaches some criterion, e.g. achieving eight correct responses in a row. We have been able to use such a system to study reversal learning in humans. Stereotyped responding in schizophrenics has been studied using a similar system with random stimuli being presented by a Pet microcomputer (Frith and Done, 1983). Many traditional psychological tests are now available for administration by microcomputer (e.g. Bexley–Maudsley psychological screening battery, NFER, Windsor, Berks.). Add-on modules are also available which enable microcomputers to sample and store psychophysiological data (e.g. skin conductance, heart rate, EEG). With these modules the computer can readily be programmed to present the subject with stimuli while at the same time recording psychophysiological data.

7.2.2 *Control of continuous processes*
The ability of computers to control processes is being used by many manufacturers to replace dedicated purpose-built controllers with cheap flexible microcomputers. For example, many liquid chromatography systems use a mixture of two different solvents which must be varied with time. Several systems available use microcomputers to monitor and adjust the concentration of each solvent in the mixture (for example Gilson and ACS market systems using an Apple II microcomputer as its controller). Some manufacturers are able to offer a choice between a dedicated controller with limited functions or a more flexible microcomputer-controlled system. For example, Actimat behavioural activity meters may be used either with their own controller or with a Commodore micro-computer.

7.2.3 *Data capture*
As implied by its name, data capture involves the recording of information during the progress of an experiment, which will involve monitoring continuous or categorical variables at specified points in time. This 'on-line' collection of new data should be distinguished from entering previously recorded data into the machine. Data can be saved for later analysis. It is also common for a certain amount of immediate analysis to occur, the results of which are stored for further analysis.

7.2.3.1 *Collection of categorical data.* An example of the use of the computer in capture of categorical data would be the collection of behavioural data from marmosets (see Chapter 2). We have successfully used a Commodore 4032 microcomputer for logging behavioural observations (Annett *et al.*, 1983; S.J. Gamble and R.M. Ridley, in preparation). Microcomputers have also been used by others (Commodore 4032 by Hendrie and Bennett, 1983; Tandy III by Depaulis, 1983); other

machines are also suitable. Our computer is programmed to record behavioural categories as previously described by Scraggs and Ridley (1979) for a manual method. The observational set-up is shown in Fig. 7.1. Observations are made through a one-way mirror. The observer presses a key on the computer keyboard to enter a code corresponding to the animal's behaviour in response to a bleep from the computer. These bleeps are emitted from the machine at accurately timed intervals, e.g. each second, and the machine collects data for a specified number of seconds. (It is usual when using a computer to type a line of data followed by a carriage return. Clearly such a system is not suitable for this rapid real-time data capture. Fortunately, many microcomputers possess a GET or INKEY command which allows the machine to accept one character of input without the need to press carriage return.) If an observer is concentrating on the animal being observed, he or she may accidentally press the wrong key. As far as possible these silly responses should be trapped by the machine and prevented from stopping the program with possible loss of data. Often the small machine used for data capture will not be used for the detailed analysis. Data should be stored in a well-defined format on to tape or floppy disk for later transfer and analysis. It is often reassuring to see the raw data printed out on paper as well, in case the tape becomes accidentally erased or overwritten.

Extra facilities can readily be written into the data capture program to allow an indication of which animals still require to have data collected, to do simple statistics such as means and standard deviations for each behaviour for each group of animals, and to do appropriate statistical tests for each behaviour between animals in different treatment groups. These functions are built into our own program for behavioural observation.

We have used several commercially available programs to transfer data from our Commodore microcomputers to our Digital main computer. Particularly successful have been Cortex Computers' 'Communicator 1' package (Commodore Business Machines, Slough) and also Les Laws' Popsys package (ANCAR (Computer Consultants) Ltd). Popsys is very flexible, allowing several microcomputers to talk to each other as well as communicating with Contact Precision Instruments' range of psychophysiology modules, or with a mainframe computer.

7.2.3.2 *Collection of continuous data.* An example of this is provided by the chromatography control systems already mentioned. The Apple II computer is also used to record the continuous output from the chromatographic detector(s). This analogue output is recorded in digital form and immediately processed to obtain peak retention times, which are printed out with an analogue record as the chromatogram. The recorded

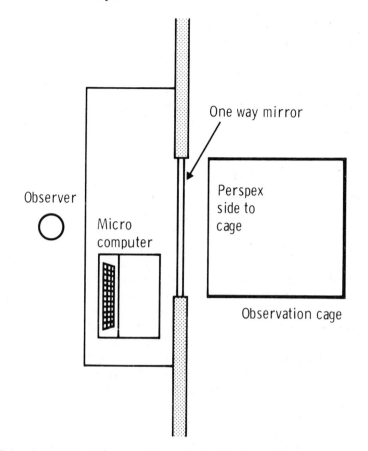

One way mirror

Observer

Micro computer

Perspex side to cage

Observation cage

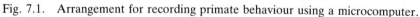

Fig. 7.1. Arrangement for recording primate behaviour using a microcomputer.

data can then be reanalysed at any time using an integration program to obtain peak heights or areas, to vary baseline correction, etc. Further calculation such as peak ratios or identification and quantification of components by comparison with standards can also be performed.

The analogue output from the chromatograph is converted into digital form by an analogue-to-digital (A-to-D) converter. A wide range of these are available for different applications, specified by sampling rate and resolution. For slowly changing voltages it is only necessary to use an A-to-D that samples the voltage a few times per second (e.g. 50 samples per second). Rapidly changing voltages will need to be monitored by a higher-speed (more samples per second) A-to-D converter. The resolution of a converter is determined by how many digital bits it has available to represent the analogue voltage. For example, if the maximum analogue voltage output from the chromatograph is +2·560 V, an 8-bit A-to-D converter is able to represent this by 2^8 (or 256) equal steps. Therefore the resolution (minimum change in voltage that would be represented as a change in digital output) would be 10 mV. An A-to-D with a resolution of 12 bits is able to represent this same voltage by 2^{12} (or 4096) equal steps and therefore has a resolution of $10/2^4 = 0.625$ mV.

7.3 Data storage and analysis

7.3.1 *Record keeping*

Data storage and processing using a computer are not different in any logical way, in terms of what is being done, from conventional laboratory record keeping. The keyboard, the VDU (visual display unit) and the memory files are direct analogues of the typewriter, the paper record and the filing cabinets. The advantages of the computer system lie in the ability to correct files immediately as data are inserted, or to locate files for subsequent access or updating, or statistical analysis of results.

As well as handling text (i.e. acting like a clever typewriter) the computer is able to function as a calculator. On a calculator you may press a single button to make it carry out a pre-programmed procedure to calculate the mean, or do a *t*-test on a previously entered group of numbers. The computer works in the same way except that the number of programs available will be much larger and they will be called up by name. Just as you might write down the result in a notebook for later reference, so the computer can save the result for later use.

Another important function of the computer is to act as the laboratory filing cabinet. A large filing cabinet will have several drawers, each of which may belong to a different user. Likewise a large computer will have its storage space divided into 'drawers', each one belonging to a different user. These drawers are referred to as user directories. Just as in the filing cabinet the user directory can only hold so much, it too has fixed dimensions. In the classical paper filing system data are written on to pages, then placed in a file. These files are then given a name which reflects their content before they are placed in a logical sequence in the drawer of a filing cabinet. Pieces of paper placed in these files may carry 200 or 300 words or only one or two.

The computer situation directly parallels the paper filing system. Data from a given experiment or the text of, say, this chapter, is stored in a named computer file. Many computers organise the material they store within files into computer pages. One of these pages may contain several hundred words or only a few. As with a hand-written page the page occupies the same amount of space whether it has 10 words or 1000 words.

There are many commercially available packages for the filing of information. Often these packages include facilities to extract subsets rapidly from the stored information, e.g. the ability to list all patients with the name Smith. The most complex of these data filing systems are called database management systems (DBMS or database). We have used the RAPPORT system (Logica, Newman Street, London W1). This is available for many machines, and versions may be used on both mainframes and microcomputers. It is important to realise that any computer system is not a magic box and will not organise totally disorganised files, any more than a new filing cabinet will spontaneously organise paper information.

So far in this chapter we have referred to storing information about tests or patients in computer files. Within a file there may be a number of pages. These pages could be thought of as large tables with subjects' names down the left-hand side and different tests going across the top. A line taken from this table would show a subject's name followed by the results for that subject on each of the tests. Such a line extracted from a table would constitute a record, a collection of all the data relating to one subject. This section will consider how such records should be kept, in what physical form and how to reduce unauthorised access.

As previously noted, records can be kept in a variety of forms varying not only in the information kept but also in the physical material on which it is stored. Thus in addition to paper sheets (in files or in a fixed order in books) or magnetic code (on discs or tape in a computer), data can be stored on file cards, which may be edge-punched, microfilm, computer punched cards or paper tape. Whatever medium the records are stored on, information should ideally be under the control of one person. This not only reduces the amount of duplication but also increases security (see below).

The storage of information presents its own problems: store too much, it is difficult to access; too little and vital information could be omitted. In many instances it will be necessary to prepare a summary of the essential features of the case, and also a history of treatment. In addition, all original documents could be microfilmed and would therefore be available if any further information were required. To speed access these records would need to be indexed. A computer system could hold a brief summary of each case and the index to the microfilm. When the original (source) documents are required, the computer can search the microfilm using codes at the edges of the film frame. This is referred to as CAR (computer-aided retrieval) of microfilm. Several different manufacturers have systems available but it should be remembered that the cost involved will be quite high. Whatever system is applied, it will be necessary to use systematic information collection; random data will not miraculously fall into some kind of order.

7.3.1.1 *Data security within computer systems.* Security is important on two levels. The first level of security is the need to keep duplicate copies of information. With storage in any medium there is the possibility of loss of, or damage to, the original records. Computerised data may be lost because magnetic tapes become erased or floppy discs become warped so they cannot be read. Therefore 'back-up' copies should be kept of everything stored in a computer, just as they should be for paper files. This is done automatically in many mainframe computer systems.

The second level of security is that which controls access to the data. Prevention of unauthorised access is particularly important with information about patients. Should patient records be borrowed from other hospitals it will be necessary to inform the medical records officer concerned about the nature of the copying and who will have access to it; he will need to be assured of confidentiality before releasing information. It is important, but fortunately relatively easy, to maintain security (i.e. confidentiality) of data stored in computer systems. If information is written on paper, it is easily available to unauthorised people. Information on a computer disc already requires some additional knowledge before the information can be read. With a large time-sharing system (a large computer used by many people at the same time) a password is usually required before an individual's files can be accessed.

Unless absolutely necessary the patient's name and address should be left out of the computer system. All information can be identified by a patient code number which matches a list of names stored elsewhere. If it is necessary to store the patient's name, this can be stored in a file separate from the rest of the information. A program would be used to recall the name and information from both files and match them up. This recall program could also ask the user for an additional password before it would recall any data.

An additional aid to security of the information would be to codify it, a kind of temporary jumbling up. Most of the database management systems have the ability to do this built in. If you write your own programs, it is fairly easy to write your own routines to codify data. Each character, be it a letter, number or symbol, is stored as a number by the computer. The most common form of code used is the ASCII system (American Standard Code for Information Interchange). All computers using ASCII use the same numbers to represent the same characters. A convenient way to code the data would be, for instance, to add the length of the password to the number representing each character in the information to be stored. Our computer might store the number 64 to represent the letter A, 65 for B, etc. If the password we choose has a length of four characters, then for the letter A the computer would store 68 (64 + 4) which normally represents the character E. Anybody attempting to read the information without using a recall program which subtracted 4 from each coded value before reconversion would find the character E, and thus the file would be unintelligible.

In considering computerised patient information systems, account also needs to be taken of the data protection acts introduced recently in various countries. It is a common requirement that details of what information is being stored, on which people and for what purposes are registered with a database registrar (although no such registration is required for keeping easily accessible hand- or typewritten files!). Some countries, e.g. Sweden, specifically forbid the inclusion of names and addresses in computer databases except in exceptional circumstances.

7.3.2 *Data processing*

Many laboratory instruments provide results in the form of lists of numbers, for example the optical densities of different solutions, or counts per minute from a scintillation counter. Some kind of formula must be applied to these figures to determine, for example, the exact amount of protein in a solution or how much drug binds to a receptor site. These sorts of small calculations are ideal tasks for computers.

It is fairly easy for the computer to deal with more complex calculations. For example, in ligand binding assays the manual calculation of the affinity of binding of a drug to its receptor by the method of Scatchard (1949, see also Chapter 6 section 6.7.1) can be fairly time consuming yet can be achieved in a few seconds using a simple computer program (see Appendix 7.1). Having calculated the initial results, the computer has the facility to store them for later more extensive analysis (cf. the laboratory filing cabinet).

Another application of the microcomputer that we have already discussed is the collection of coded data on animal (or human) behaviour. In addition to the simple tabulation of time spent on each category of behaviour, the computer can calculate the number of changes of behaviour in a given time, length of run of each behaviour and transition matrices. A transition matrix analyses which behaviour preceded the current behaviour: e.g. in a given period how many times does behaviour 1 precede behaviour 2? Second order transition matrices can also be calculated: i.e. what are the two behaviours immediately preceding the current behaviour? Caution is necessary, however, since the number of possible combinations may become large in relation to the numbers of observations made, so that unrepresentative samples are obtained. Further details of the analysis of behavioural sequences is given by Lewis and Gower (1980). Some of the methods involve the application of information theory techniques to behavioural information. This subject is discussed extensively by Attneave (1959). (Many of the methods used for looking at patterns in behaviour are similar to those used for modelling patterns in DNA sequences. The journal *Nucleic Acids Research* (1984) has devoted a whole issue to this problem.)

Tabulations of results held in the computer are immediately available for statistical analysis, using the type of package mentioned at the end of the introduction. Minitab in particular lends itself to data tabulation and relatively straightforward analysis. Other packages, e.g. PSTAT (P-STAT Inc., New Jersey, USA), are able to carry out tabulation and more complex statistical analysis, but are harder to use. The purpose of the rest of this chapter is to provide guidelines on the selection and use of suitable tests to determine the statistical significance of the results obtained.

7.4 Data examination and statistical methods

7.4.1 *Introduction*
It is obviously impossible to give full details of many statistical procedures in the short space available here. We have therefore restricted ourselves to naming procedures and describing the conditions in which they should be used, with some examples. A summary of tests and conditions is given in Appendix 2. Armed with this information the intrepid reader should be able to find the necessary details in statistical textbooks or in the manuals of statistics packages for computers.

Take statistical advice before you collect your data, not after. It is advisable to select the type of statistical analysis you are going to use before you start to collect the data. When making decisions of this sort it would be extremely useful to have the advice of an expert on statistical analysis and experimental design. For example it is crucial to ascertain before starting an experiment that the design will actually permit the testing of the hypothesis of interest. It is also possible to estimate in advance the number of subjects that will be needed to reject or accept the hypothesis unequivocally. This is done on the basis of the likely size of the experimental effect and on the variability of the measures being used (Altman, 1980).

7.4.2 *Inter-observer agreement*
For a general discussion of inter-observer agreement the reader is directed to Berk (1979). Before processing the data we have collected, we need to have some assurance that we have actually measured what we intended to measure and that we have measured it accurately. This may seem the consequence of unnecessary and even foolish doubts, particular-

ly if laboratory-based procedures have been used. Even here we need some check on the consistency of our measures. This problem is discussed in various other sections of this book in relation to specific laboratory techniques. However, in the study of psychiatric disorders many measures are not laboratory based. For example, we might wish to assess the severity of movement disorders or hallucinations. There is clearly the possibility in such assessments that different observers will assess different things or will change their criteria of severity. Even with a highly technical procedure such as computerised axial tomography, the final measure might be a visual assessment of the overall abnormality of the scan which could also be subject to observer differences and biases. In all these cases it is very important to have some index of whether something is actually being measured and measured accurately.

The most straightforward way of making such a check is to have the same measures made by two independent observers. If there is a close agreement between the observers, then we may be more confident that something is being measured and that it is being measured accurately. If the measurement is continuous, and normally distributed, then the Pearson product moment correlation would be appropriate (see section 7.4.4.1(d)). However, it is more likely with this type of rating that a very crude ordinal scale will be used; for example movement disorders might be rated as severe, mild or non-existent. In this case the relationship between the two raters can be assessed from the contingency table shown in Table 7.1. Here the subjects have been divided into four groups on the basis of A's ratings and one can ask whether these groups differ significantly in terms of B's ratings. This can be done using analysis of variance by ranks (Meddis, 1980), and the relevant cases will be discussed in section 7.4.4.2(a). Since we expect a linear relationship between the two raters (by analogy with the linear regression in the correlation used for parametric data), we can apply a *post-hoc* trend analysis (Page, 1963). This reveals a highly significant relationship between the two raters.

In many cases the scales may not be ordinal, but only categorical. For example, two diagnosticians might classify patients as schizophrenic, depressive or neurotic. A contingency table similar to that shown in Table 7.1 can still be drawn up, but now the data cannot be ranked and thus a test based on frequency and on the χ^2 must be used (section 7.4.4.2(d)). A significant χ^2 associated with such a table will indicate any consistent relationship between the two diagnosticians, but this might indicate that patients classified as schizophrenic by one rater were classified as depressed by the other. Partitioning of the χ^2 statistics (Maxwell, 1961) should give a more specific test of the extent to which the raters not only divide the patients into the same groups, but also give the groups the same labels.

A significant statistic indicates that the two observers are measuring

Table 7.1.   Inter-rater reliability. 40 patients rated for hallucinations on a four-point scale by two observers. The table shows the number of patients rated in all the possible ways by the two observers.

		Rater A		
Rater B	*None*	*Possible*	*Mild*	*Severe*
None	3	1	0	0
Possible	3	2	1	0
Mild	2	11	5	0
Severe	1	3	4	4

Rater B's scores were compared for the four groups of patients defined by rater A's scores (Kruskal–Wallace test — Siegel, 1956). Overall comparison: $\chi^2 = 13.4$, df $= 3$, $P < 0.01$. Linear component: $z = 3.67$, $P < 0.001$. There is significant agreement between the two observers.

something in common. If the statistic is not significant, then nothing useful is being measured and the measure should be revised and made more concrete. It is also possible to train observers until they reach agreement about what they are observing. However, this does not seem too useful unless they can subsequently specify what they have agreed about so that the same technique can be used by other people.

Even if there is a significant relationship between observers there can still be systematic differences between them. For example, if one observer constantly gave more severe ratings than the other, a strong relationship would still result (see Table 7.2).

A systematic difference of this sort between observers would not matter if the ratings from both observers were to be combined or if the ratings from only one observer were to be used. However, if, in the final study, some patients were rated by one observer and some by the other, then apparent differences in severity between patients might in fact be the consequence of systematic differences between the raters. It is clearly important to take such a possibility into account when different patients are rated by different people.

7.4.3 *Data examination and cleansing*
Once the data have been stored in the computer the most important and time-consuming activity to be carried out before any statistical analysis is 'data cleansing'. This has the purpose of identifying any mistakes and oddities and suggesting what sort of statistical analyses will be most appropriate. Data cleansing is best carried out by plotting the data in various ways. Tukey (1977) describes a great many useful ways of looking at data.

Table 7.2. Inter-rater differences. 40 patients rated for hallucinations by two observers (the same data as in Table 7.1). The table shows the frequencies of the different ratings used by the two observers.

| | | Severity of symptom | | |
	None	Possible	Mild	Severe
Rater A	9	17	10	4
Rater B	4	6	18	12

Comparison of severity of ratings (Mann–Whitney test — Siegel, 1956). $z = 3.40$, $P < 0.001$. Rater B rates symptoms systematically more severely than rater A.

7.4.3.1 *Histograms.* It is essential to plot histograms of the data for each of the groups or conditions to be compared. Such plots show how many subjects have any particular value of the relevant variable. For example on a rating scale ten subjects might have a score of 0, five subjects a score of 1, and so on. Continuous variables such as hormone levels can be split up into bands of values to give exactly the same type of plot. In most cases a histogram plotting program will handle this aspect of the plot automatically. Such plots frequently reveal outliers. These are points which clearly stand apart from the main bulk of the distribution (Fig. 7.2). A useful rule of thumb defines outliers as being at least two standard deviations away from the mean of the distribution (i.e. the well known, but arbitrary, less than 5% probability of occurring by chance).

The most likely cause of outliers is a mistake in data entry. Thus a number punched in the wrong column might give a value of 800 instead of 8. These mistakes can be rectified by going back to the original source of the data. Inclusion of such erroneous values in the statistical analyses can easily give rise to misleading results, particularly when correlation is involved.

If the outlier does not arise from faulty data entry, it is possible that the original value has been derived incorrectly. For example, if the value has been derived from a Scatchard analysis, the analysis should be checked.

Unfortunately it is sometimes the case that the outlying value cannot be identified as an error. For some, possibly unknown, reason that subject just has a very deviant value. In order that sensible parametric statistics can be carried out it is necessary to leave that subject out of all subsequent analyses. However, it is obviously important to take careful note of who is being left out and why. If it is considered essential to retain these deviant values, then non-parametric statistics can be used since they use ranks or frequencies rather than absolute values.

The histogram plot also gives a rough idea of how normal is the shape of the distribution. This is important in deciding on the most appropriate

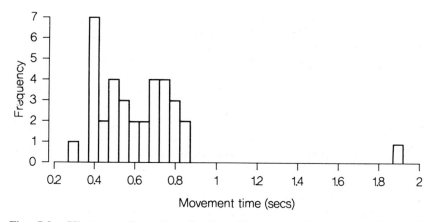

Fig. 7.2. Histogram Revealing Outlier. Histogram of movement times (in seconds) showing an outlier two standard deviations beyond the mean (mean = 0.59, SD = 0.28).

statistical tests. For the more versatile parametric tests the distribution must be roughly normal. In other words most subjects must have values in the middle of the range with fewer subjects having values above or below these medium values as in Fig. 7.3. In some cases, particularly with scores coming from rating scales, the distributions will clearly be skewed so that, for example, most subjects will have scores of 0 with progressively fewer subjects having higher scores (Fig. 7.4). With such distributions parametric statistics cannot normally be used.

7.4.3.2 Normal probability plots (Royston, 1982). Normal probability plots provide a convenient method for looking at the shape of a distribution of scores and, in particular, for checking for normality. However, such plots are only practicable if there is an appropriate computer program available. For parametric statistics to be applicable to a set of data the residuals should be normally distributed. The residual is the difference between the predicted and the observed value of an observation. For simple analyses such as group comparisons the predicted value of an observation is simply the mean of the group from which that observation comes. Thus in order to put more than one group on the same plot it is necessary first to subtract the group mean from each score. To construct a normal probability plot the residual scores from all the subjects are first put into rank order. Given the rank of an individual score and knowing the mean and SD of the total distribution it is possible to estimate the value that a score of that rank ought to have if the distribution were normal. A plot of the predicted against the observed values will then give

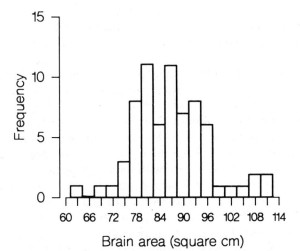

Fig. 7.3. Histogram of normally distributed data. Histogram of cross-sectional brain area in a group of schizophrenic patients. The distribution is roughly normal.

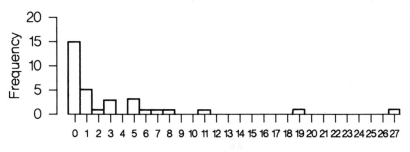

Fig. 7.4. Histogram of non-normally distributed data. Histogram of the number of rest pauses taken by patients during a 90-s tapping task. The distribution is far from normal since most subjects took no rest pauses. These data will have to be analysed non-parametrically.

a straight line if the distribution were indeed normal. Presented in this form departures from normality in the data are relatively easy to observe. A test for the normality of the distribution based on the correlation between observed and predicted scores is also available (Royston, 1982). Many program packages will derive normal probability plots and Minitab and SPP also give tests of significance.

Outliers will also be revealed in normal plots as a few points at either end of the line which deviate from the linearity of the other points (Fig. 7.5). Such points must be investigated and dealt with as described in section 7.4.3.1.

Instead of being linear the normal probability plot may form some kind of smooth curve (Fig. 7.6a). Most commonly a negatively accelerating curve is observed. A smooth curve of this type suggests that a transformation can be found that will normalise the data. A normal probability plot of the transformed data will then give a straight line. The most commonly applied transformation is logarithmic ($x' = \log (x)$, Fig. 7.6b). This is frequently found to be necessary with data such as hormone levels, drug levels and time scores (e.g. reaction times). Other and more complex transformation may be necessary with other kinds of data, but for these it would probably be best to take statistical advice. If a statistics package is available, it is easy to try normal probability plots on different transformations of the data to see if any will successfully normalise them.

If the normal plot is neither linear nor shows a smooth curve, then parametric statistics probably cannot be applied and different approaches will be needed that we shall describe in a later section. This situation is particularly likely to arise when the data comes from rating scales (ordinal) or counts of things such as number of symptoms or number of episodes.

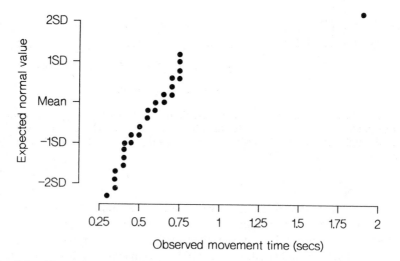

Fig. 7.5. Normal probability plot revealing outlier. Normal probability plot of the data shown in Fig. 7.2. The outlier is clearly revealed.

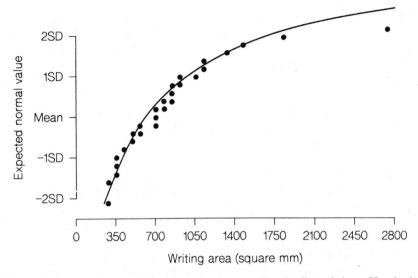

Fig. 7.6a. Normal probability plot of non-normally distributed data. Handwriting area was measured in patients who were subsequently given neuroleptic drugs. The normal probability plot clearly shows a systematic deviation from normality. Thus the raw scores are not normally distributed.

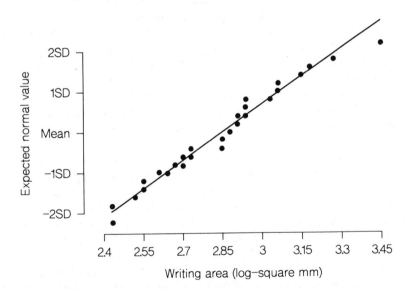

Fig. 7.6b. Normal probability plot of data normalised by transformation. The data shown in Fig. 7.6a were transformed into logs. The normal probability plot is now clearly linear. The data have been normalised by this transformation.

7.4.4 *Statistical analysis*

Statistical analysis of data is an enormous and complicated subject which is well beyond the scope of this book let alone this section of this chapter. We shall confine ourselves to describing very briefly some basic tests that may be used in commonly occurring situations and pointing out some problems and pitfalls.

7.4.4.1 *Parametric tests.* These are powerful and versatile tests that should certainly be used if the data have passed the tests of normality described in section 7.4.3.2.

(a) *Analysis of variance (Winer, 1971).* This technique can be applied to test for differences between two or more groups (e.g. cross-sectional brain area in schizophrenia, affective disorders and Alzheimer's disease). The resultant statistic is the F-ratio. The independent t-test is a special case of analysis of variance applied to only two groups. In this case the F-ratio is the square of the t-value. Descriptions of the theory and methodology of analysis of variance can be found in any textbook of statistics. In essence the method asks the question, 'Is the variance between the groups greater than the variance within the groups?' If it is, then the groups must be considered to have different means. Clearly problems will arise if the variances of the individual groups differ to any great extent. This 'homogeneity of variance' should certainly be checked for and it would be as well to take advice if the SD of one group was more than double that of another. Statistics packages such as BMDP and SPP frequently do a test for homogeneity of variance and may even provide alternative statistics which are not affected by unequal variances. Although it is convenient to have equal numbers within groups, unequal numbers do not constitute a problem as long as there is only one factor along which the groups are classified (e.g. diagnostic categories). Table 7.3 shows the results of a one-way analysis of variance.

(b) *Analysis of variance with more than one way of classifying the groups.* If the groups can be classified along more than one dimension (e.g. diagnosis, sex, age), this should be taken advantage of in an analysis of variance, which is then called two- (or more) way ANOVA, as opposed to one-way ANOVA discussed in section 7.4.4.1(a). It is possible to look at the effect of each dimension independently, and to see if there is any interaction between them. The technique can also provide a means of eliminating the effects of confounding variables such as sex. For example brain area might be measured in various diagnostic groups. This measure is believed to be influenced by the sex of the subject. We can divide the diagnostic groups into male and female and carry out a two-way analysis

Table 7.3.   One-way analysis of variance (ANOVA). Cross-sectional brain areas
were measured for three types of patient.

	n	Mean (cm^2)	Standard deviation (SD)
Schizophrenic	26	83.94	9.32
Affective	21	83.78	9.06
Alzheimer's	17	77.37	10.90

Homogeneity of variance (largest variance over smallest) $= \left(\dfrac{10.90}{9.06}\right)^2 = 1.45$, ns

ANOVA table Source of variance	Degrees of freedom (df)	Sum of squares (SS)	Mean square (MS)	F-ratio	Probability
Between groups	2	527.5	263.8	2.82	< 0.07
Within groups	61	5714	93.7		
Total	63	6242			

of variance. This will reveal whether there is a significant effect of sex, whether there is a significant effect of diagnosis independent of sex, and also whether there is an interaction between the two dimensions (see Table 7.4). A significant interaction would indicate, for example, that there was a difference in brain weight between female schizophrenics and female controls, but not between male schizophrenics and male controls. It is clear that if the interaction is significant, then interpretation of any significant main effects must take the interaction into account. A plot of the relevant mean values is often extremely helpful in interpreting interactions. In the case of two-way analysis, if a simple ANOVA is being used, then the groups of subjects should be roughly equal or at least proportional. If this is not the case, it would be best to take advice. Packages such as BMDP use methods that overcome the problem of unequal groups.

(c) *Repeated measures*. Often the same subject will be measured more than once. This raises problems since two scores from the same subject are clearly not independent, and independence is one of the prime requirements of most statistical tests (including non-parametric ones). This problem can be overcome if there is some way of reducing the scores of each subject to a single score. If only two measures are involved, this can easily be achieved by using difference or ratio scores. Which of these is chosen will depend on the nature of the data and the shape of its distribution. The logs of ratio scores are of course identical to difference scores of logarithmically transformed data. The correlated or related

Table 7.4.   Two-way analysis of variance. Cross-sectional brain areas for three types of patient subdivided by sex (the same data as in Table 7.3).

	n	Female mean	SD	n	Male mean	SD	Means for diagnosis
Schizophrenic	16	81.37	8.61	9	89.43	8.78	84.27
Affective	14	81.33	8.14	7	88.69	9.38	83.78
Alzheimer's	7	67.84	6.79	9	84.64	8.00	77.29
Means for sex		78.8			87.5		

Homogeneity of variance (largest variance over smallest) $= \left(\dfrac{9.38}{6.79}\right)^2 = 1.91$, ns

ANOVA table

Source	df	MS	F	P
Diagnosis	2	501.6	7.19	< 0.01
Sex	1	1617	23.18	< 0.0001
Diagnosis × sex	2	129.3	1.85	ns
Within groups	56	69.76		
Total	61	101.5		

A large sex difference is revealed and the difference between diagnostic groups is enhanced in comparison with Table 7.3. This is in part because there were relatively more males in the Alzheimer's group.

t-test is a special case of this technique in which difference scores for a single group of subjects are compared with zero. For example, a group of subjects perform a motor-skill test twice with a 5-min rest between the two occasions. We wish to know whether they have improved their performance. We therefore find the difference between the two occasions for each subject and test whether these differences are significantly greater than zero, i.e. no change. When the data from a subject have been reduced to a single score, then the methods of group comparison described above can be used. With more than two conditions, e.g. repeated testing over time (Fig. 7.7), matters become more complicated and advice should be taken. Transformations to trends or orthogonal polynomials are often useful, but are well beyond the scope of this section (Edwards, 1968, Chapter 14). It is also possible to perform multivariate analysis of variance (MANOVA).

(d) *Correlation and regression (Draper and Smith, 1968)*. These techniques for investigating the relationship between variables will be described in any textbook of statistics. However, they raise a number of problems and should be used with caution. Many statistics packages will carry out linear and higher order regressions, but it is desirable to have, in

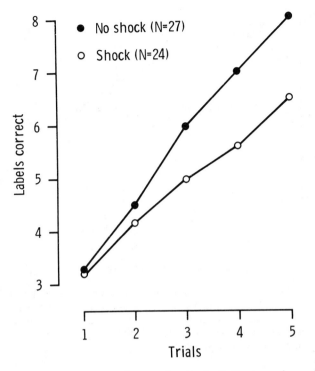

Fig. 7.7. Learning data suitable for trend analysis. Patients performed a learning task (learning labels for faces) after real or sham ECT. There were five trials per subject and so a repeated measures ANOVA would be appropriate. The learning clearly takes the form of a linear improvement over trials. Calculation of *linear trends* would considerably simplify the analysis of these data.

advance, a hypothesis about the exact relationship between the two variables. For example it has been claimed that there is a curvilinear relationship between brain weight and age, such that loss of brain weight is more rapid after the age of 50. This can be tested by fitting a quadratic regression line to the data (Fig. 7.8).

(e) *Covariance analysis (Winer, 1971)*. This provides a means of eliminating confounding variables such as age from group comparisons (Table 7.5). This technique should also be used with caution. The groups to be compared should have a considerable overlap in terms of the variable to be covaried out. If the groups differed markedly on age, then the results of the covariance analysis would be extremely artificial since the technique depends essentially on predicting what the subjects would have been like if they had all had the same age. This should not involve extrapolation outside the range of the data available. It is also required that the

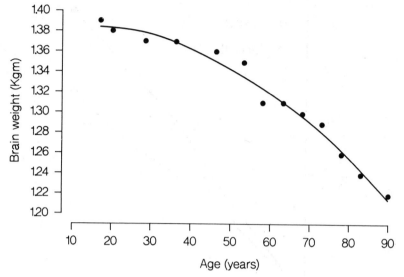

Fig. 7.8. Variables showing a curvilinear relationship. A curvilinear relationship is hypothesised to exist between brain weight and age (data from Dekaban and Sadowsky, 1978). Quadratic regression gives a very good fit with the following parameters: weight $= 1.4 + 0.0007$ (age) $- 0.00003$ (age)^2. Both the linear and quadratic components were significant.

relationship between age and the dependent variable should be the same in all groups. In the case of major differences in ages between the groups, it would clearly be better to go back and collect some more comparable subjects.

7.4.4.2 *Non-parametric tests (Siegel, 1956).* If the data are not distributed normally, then non-parametric tests have to be used. These fall into two major divisions: those using raw scores as in the parametric tests (but replacing these raw scores by ranks) and those using frequencies or counts. Within these categories there are large numbers of tests all developed for slightly different purposes. It is impossible to describe them all here. Meddis's (1980) paper on unified analysis of variance by ranks has improved the situation considerably by showing that many non-parametric tests are special cases of this one method. Our presentation of non-parametric methods of data analysis has been strongly influenced by Meddis's approach to the problem. Whether it is appropriate to use raw scores or frequencies will depend partly on the distribution of the data and partly on the nature of the measure. If too many subjects have the same value, then frequencies will probably have to be used. For example, half the subjects in a sample might have a zero rating on a scale of

Table 7.5. Covariance analysis. Covariance analysis (ANCOVA) of cross-sectional brain area for schizophrenic patients with or without defect state.

	Intact n = 50	Defect state n = 25
Age (years)	67.0	73.8
Brain area (cm²)	89.1	85.4
Brain area corrected for age	88.0	86.3

There is a considerable difference in the age of the two types of patient as well as in brain area. When this difference in age is allowed for by covariance analysis, the difference in brain area is much reduced.

movement disorder. In this case it might well be better to use frequencies dividing the subjects into those with and those without movement disorders. If the measure is nominal (e.g. schizophrenic, affective, demented) rather than ordinal (e.g. normal, mild, severe), then frequency scores must obviously be used. For example we might count the number of subjects in the sample who have the diagnosis of schizophrenia, or manic depression or dementia. Using data of this kind it is important that each subject can only appear in one category (e.g. a demented schizophrenic cannot appear in both categories). If a subject appears in more than one category, then the assumption of independence between categories is violated and statistical analysis becomes very tricky.

(a) *Group comparisons using raw scores.* Two groups can be compared using the Mann–Whitney U-test (equivalent to the uncorrelated t-test) and more than two groups by using the Kruskal–Wallace test. All the scores are first ranked, ignoring group memberships, and then mean ranks for the various groups are calculated. If the groups are ordered or can be classified in more than one way, then the equivalents of main effects and interactions in the analysis of variance (sections 7.4.4.1(a) and (b)) can be calculated by using Page's test for trends (Page, 1963) (Table 7.6).

(b) *Comparisons using frequencies (Maxwell, 1961; Everitt, 1977).* If there are relatively few possible scores (e.g. 1, 2, 3 = normal, mild, severe), it is more convenient to present the data as a frequency table (e.g. Table 7.7). However, as long as the data are ordinal (as in this example), then ranking methods can still be used to compare the groups.

Groups for which only nominal data are available may be compared using the χ^2 test (using Yates' correction) unless the cell sizes are very small in which case Fisher's exact test should be used. When there are

Table 7.6. Non-parametric group comparisons (raw scores). Group comparisons, individual subject data on an ordinal measure (Kruskal-Wallace test). 4 groups of patients were treated with different drug regimes and rated for movement disorder on a 4-point scale (0 = none; 1 = possible; 2 = mild; 3 = severe). All of the data were ranked ignoring group membership.

										Mean rank
Group 1 (placebo)	$n = 5$:	raw data:	0	1	0	1	2			
		ranks:	3	9.5	3	9.5	17			8.4
Group 2 (neuroleptics)	$n = 7$:	raw data:	1	2	3	2	3	2	2	
		ranks:	9.5	17	22	17	22	17	17	17.4
Group 3 (anti-cholinergic)	$n = 6$:	raw data:	0	1	1	1	1	3		
		ranks:	3	9.5	9.5	9.5	9.5	22		10.5
Group 4 (neuroleptic + anti-cholinergic)	$n = 5$:	raw data:	0	2	0	1	2			
		ranks:	3	17	3	9.5	17			9.9

Overall difference between groups: $\chi^2 = 7.13$, df = 3, $P < 0.07$. Main effects (neuroleptic vs no neuroleptic, anti-cholinergic vs no anti-cholinergic) and interactions were assessed with Page's test. Interaction: $z = 3.39$, $P < 0.06$. Thus there is a tendency for neuroleptics to increase movement disorders, but not if given in conjunction with anti-cholinergics.

more than two groups, various procedures for partitioning the χ^2 test are available which make possible comparisons analogous to main effects and interactions in analysis of variance (Table 7.7).

(c) *Repeated measures.* If the underlying data are not normally distributed, then repeated measures present considerable problems. As stated in section 7.4.4.1(b), it is desirable to manipulate the data to give a single measure for each subject. The obvious choice is to use difference scores. However, to calculate difference scores and then use non-parametric statistics (e.g. Wilcoxon test) does not entirely overcome the problem since the act of calculating difference scores may already be making unjustifiable assumptions about the data. In particular we are assuming that a change in symptom severity (for example) from 4 to 2 is the same as a change from 2 to 0. If this sort of assumption is in doubt, then all we can look at is whether the score increases, remains unchanged or goes down. In this case we are converting our scores to frequency data (e.g. ten subjects got worse, two got better). For such data a sign test may be used to look at changes within a single group (equivalent to a matched pairs *t*-test) and a χ^2 test may be used to compare groups as in section 7.4.4.2(b). With more than two repeated measures it is possible to rank conditions within each subject and use Friedman's test to see if there are significant differences between conditions. Once again if conditions can

Table 7.7. Non-parametric group comparisons (frequencies). Group comparisons, frequency data on an ordinal measure. Three categories of chronic schizophrenic patient with ventricle sizes rated as small, medium or large. All the data were ranked ignoring group membership.

Ventricle size (rank)	Small (16.5)	Medium (49)	Large (88)	Mean rank
Defect state (type 2)	15	10	15	51.4
Positive symptoms (type 1)	7	7	13	59.4
Others	10	16	17	56.9

Overall group difference: $\chi^2 = 1.29$, ns

be classified in more than one way, then main effects and interactions can also be tested. However, this is only possible with one group of subjects. If there are several groups of subjects with each subject tested in a number of different conditions, then there is no simple non-parametric test which permits estimation of the groups by conditions interaction (see Table 7.8).

(d) *Correlations.* If ordinal scores are available, then Spearman's rank order correlation will overcome the problem of a lack of normality in the

Table 7.8. Non-parametric comparison of conditions. Comparison of conditions within subjects, individual scores, ordinal measure (Friedman test). Six patients treated with four different drug regimes and rated for movement disorder on a 4-point scale. This is a repeat of the experiment shown in Table 7.6 using a within-subject rather than a between-subject design. The data were ranked for each subject separately. The ranks are shown in brackets.

	Placebo	Neuroleptic	Anti-cholinergic	Neuroleptic + anti-cholinergic
Subject 1	0 (2)	1 (4)	0 (2)	0 (2)
2	1 (1.5)	2 (3.5)	1 (1.5)	1 (3.5)
3	0 (1.5)	3 (4)	1 (3)	0 (1.5)
4	1 (2)	2 (4)	1 (2)	1 (2)
5	2 (3)	3 (4)	1 (1.5)	1 (1.5)
6	2 (2)	2 (2)	3 (4)	2 (2)
Mean rank	2.0	3.6	2.3	2.1

Overall test for differences between groups; $\chi^2 = 7.98$, df $= 3$, $P < 0.05$. Main effects and interactions were assessed with Page's test. Interaction: neuroleptic × anticholinergic; $z = 4.12$, $P < 0.05$. Neuroleptics increase movement disorder when given alone, but not in conjunction with anti-cholinergics.

Table 7.9. Non-parametric test of association. Test of association using categorical data. Is there a relationship between type of psychotic symptom and type of epilepsy? The data is from Trimble and Perez (1982).

	Temporal lobe epilepsy	*Generalised epilepsy*
Schizophrenic symptoms	12	2
Manic-depressive symptoms	6	5

χ^2 (using Yates' correction) $= 1.62$, df $= 1$, ns. Fisher's exact test, $P = 0.10$

Table 7.10. Non-parametric covariance analysis. A test of partial associations using frequency data. This is analogous to analysis of covariance. Within a large group of chronic schizophrenic patients the relationships between defect state, neuroleptic treatment and length of illness were assessed. A maximum likelihood χ^2 analysis based on a log-linear model was used.

Defect state	*Neuroleptic treatment*	*Length of illness (years)*			
		< 10	$10–20$	$20–30$	> 30
	none	1	4	10	40
No	some	1	10	24	65
	a lot	19	46	78	100
	none	0	0	0	10
Yes	some	0	4	4	32
	a lot	0	9	12	41

A test of the partial associations of the factors, i.e. the effect of the third factor is removed. Length of illness × defect state: likelihood ratio $\chi^2 = 18.04$, df $= 3$, $P < 0.001$. Neuroleptic × defect state: likelihood ratio $\chi^2 = 4.14$, df $= 2$, ns. Defect state is related to length of illness, but not to neuroleptic treatment.

distributions of the two measures being related. Where frequencies only are available, then the χ^2 test gives a measure of relationship (see section 7.4.4(b). More complex non-linear relationships can also be investigated by partitioning the χ^2 test and testing for the particular trend hypothesised. (see Table 7.9)

(e) *Covariance (Plackett, 1974)*. Clearly situations may arise for frequency data in which we would like to be able to covary out the effect of some confounding variable. For example, can schizophrenic defect state be completely accounted for by length of illness, or is there an additional effect of neuroleptic medication? Such questions can be answered by using log-linear models, but these are beyond the scope of this book. It should also be borne in mind that any multivariate comparison requires many more subjects to provide an unequivocal answer than does a univariate comparison.

From the foregoing examples it can be seen that non-parametric data analysis is in many ways more difficult than parametric data analysis. Thus one should try to collect parametric data if this is possible; however, in the real world we have to analyse what we can get, as well as getting what we can analyse. Appendix 7.2 summarises appropriate tests for different types of data.

References

Alcock, D. (1977). *Illustrating Basic (a simple Programming Language)*, Cambridge University Press, Cambridge

Alcock, D. (1982). *Illustrating Fortran (The portable Variety)*, Cambridge University Press, Cambridge

Altman, D.G. (1980). How large a sample? *Brit. Med. J.* **281**, 1336–8.

Anderson, R.G. (1979). *Data Processing and Management Information Systems*, 3rd edn, Macdonald and Evans, Plymouth.

Annett, L.E., Ridley, R.M., Gamble, S.J. and Baker H.F. (1983). Behavioural effects of intracerebral amphetamine in the marmoset. *Psychopharmacol.* **81**, 18–23.

Association of Clinical Biochemists (1983). *A Guide to Data Processing in Clinical Laboratories*, Association of Clinical Biochemists, London.

Attneave, F. (1959). *Applications of Information Theory to Psychology*, Henry Holt and Company, New York.

Berk, R. (1979). Generalizability of behavioural observations: a classification of interobserver agreement and interobserver reliability. *Am.J.Mental Deficiency*, **83**, 460–72.

British Medical Journal (1983). **286**, 28 May–1 Oct.

Chandor, A. (Ed.) (1979). *Penguin Dictionary of Computers*, 2nd edn, Penguin, Harmondsworth.

Dekaben, A.S. and Sadowsky, D. (1978). Changes in brain weight during the span of human life. *Annals of Neurology*, **4**, 345–56.

Depaulis, A. (1983). A microcomputer method for behavioral data acquisition and subsequent analysis. *Pharmacol. Biochem. Behav.* **19**, 729–32.

Draper, N.R. and Smith, H. (1968). *Applied Regression Analysis*, Wiley, London.

Edwards, A.L. (1968). *Experimental Design in Psychological Research*, Holt, Rinehart & Winston, London.

Everitt, B.G. (1977). *The Analysis of Contingency Tables*, Chapman & Hall, London.

Frith, C.D. and Done, D.J. (1983). Stereotyped responding by schizophrenic patients on a two-choice guessing task. *Psychol. Med.* **13**, 779–86.

Hendrie, C.A. and Bennett, S. (1983). A microcomputer technique for the detailed analysis of animal behaviour. *Physiol. Behav.* **30**, 233–5.

Lewis, D.B. and Gower, D.M. (1980). *Biology of Communication*, Blackie, London.

Maxwell, A.R. (1961). *Analysing Qualitative Data*, Methuen, London.

Meddis, R. (1980). Unified analysis of variance by ranks. *Brit. J. Math. Stat.*

Psychol. **33**, 84–98.

Medical Laboratory Sciences (1980). **37**, No. 3, Institute of Medical Laboratory Sciences, London.

Munro, D. (1974). *Interactive Computing with Basic*, Edward Arnold, London.

Munro, D. (1975). *Interactive Computing with Fortran*, Edward Arnold, London.

Nucleic Acids Research (1984). **12**, No. 1. Parts 1 and 2, January 1984.

Page, C.B. (1963). Ordered hypothesis for multiple treatments: a significance test for linear ranks. *J. Am. Stat. Assn.* **58**, 216–30.

Parkin, A. (1975). *Cobol for Students*, Edward Arnold, London.

Plackett, R.L. (1974). *The Analysis of Categorical Data*, Griffin, London.

Royston, J.P. (1982). An extension of Shapiro and Wilk's W test for normality of large samples. *J. Royal Stat. Soc.: Series C* (Applied Statistics) **31**, 115–24.

Scatchard, G. (1949). *Ann. New York Acad. Science*, **51**, 660–72.

Scraggs, P.R. and Ridley, R.M. (1979). The effect of dopamine and noradrenaline blockade on amphetamine-induced behaviour in the marmoset. *Psychopharmacol.* **66**, 41–3.

Siegel, S. (1956). *Nonparametric Statistics for the Behavioural Sciences*, McGraw-Hill, New York.

Siemasko, F. (Ed.) (1978). *Computing in Clinical Laboratories*, Pitman Medical, Bath.

Trimble, M.R. and Perez, M.M. (1982). The phenomenology of the chronic psychoses of epilepsy. *Adv. Biol. Psychiat.*, **8**, 98–105.

Tukey, J.W. (1977). *Exploratory Data Analysis*, Addison-Wesley Reading, Mass.

Winer, B.J. (1971). *Statistical Principles in Experimental Design*, McGraw-Hill, New York.

Woolbridge, S. (1976). *Data Processing Made Simple*, W.H. Allen, London.

Appendix 7.1 An example of a simple program written in BASIC

```
00001 REM RESTART POINT
00005 GOSUB 900
00010PRINT
00012PRINT
00014PRINT
00015PRINT"        SCATCHARD PROGRAM"
00016PRINT" =============================================================="
00018PRINT
00020PRINT
00022PRINT"    DO YOU WANT INSTRUCTIONS?"
00030 INPUT A$
00040 IF A$="Y"GOTO 650
00050PRINT
00060PRINT
00070PRINT
00080PRINT
00090PRINT
00100 GOSUB 900
00110PRINT"ENTER COUNTS PER F/MOL"
00112INPUT K
00114IF K<0.1 THEN GOTO 110
00120Y=0x=0x1=0x2=0y1=0y2=0z=0a=0
00125PRINTpRINTpRINT"    HOW MANY DATA POINTS?"
00126INPUT G
00127 IF G<3  THEN GOTO 129
00128 GOTO 131
00129PRINT "NOT ENOUGH DATA POINTS !!!!!!!!!!"
00130 GOTO 125
00131 FOR J=1 TO G
00132 PRINT "DATA POINT NUMBER = "; J
00140N=0m=0
00150PRINT
00160PRINT "ENTER NONSPECIFIC COUNTS"
00170 INPUT N$
00180 IF N$="N" THEN GOTO 230
00190LET N=N+(VAL (N$))
00200 M=M+1
00210 GOTO 170
002200=0
00230 0=N/M
```

```
00240 PRINT "MEAN NSB COUNTS   ="; OpRINT
00250PRINT "ENTER TOTAL COUNTS."
00260N=0m=0
00270 INPUT N$
00280 IF N$="N" THEN GOTO 320
00290 N=N+(VAL (N$))
00300 M=M+1
00310GOTO 270
00320P=N/M
00330PRINT "MEAN OF TOTAL COUNTS = "; PpRINT
00340 Q=P-OpRINT "SPECIFIC BOUND COUNTS = ";Q
00350B=Q/KpRINT"F/MOLS BOUND    = ";B
00358 PRINT
00359L=0
00360 PRINT "ENTER F/MOLS OF LIGAND ADDED TO EACH TUBE
00362INPUT LpRINT
00370 F=L-BpBRINT"FREE LIGAND      = ";F
00380 A=(B/F) *1000
00390PRINT "BOUND/FREE        = ";A
00400 X=X+A
00410 X2=X2+(A2)
00420Y=Y+B
00430 Y2=Y2+(B2)
00440 Z=Z+(A*B)
00442PRINT"INPUT LETTER C TO CONTINUE"
00444 INPUT C$
00446 IF C$ 〈〉"C"THEN GOTO 442
00448 GOSUB 900
00450 NEXT J
00451 GOSUB 900
00452 PRINT"  *******CALCULATING CORRELATION ******"
00453GOSUB 900
00460 M=((Z-((X*Y)/G))/(Y2-((Y2)/G)))
00470 C=(Y-(X/M))/G
00480 X1=((X2-((X2)/G))/(G-1)).5
00490 Y1=((Y2-((Y2)/G))/(G-1)).5
00500 R=(M*Y1)/X1
00510 GOSUB 900
00520 PRINT "CORRELATION      = ";R
00530 PRINT"SLOPE            = ";M
00540 PRINT"B.MAX            = ";C
00550 PRINT"K.D.             = ";(-1/M)
00600 PRINTpRINT"    INPUT 'A'TO RUN PROGRAM AGAIN."
```

```
00610 INPUT A$
00620 IF A$="A" THEN GOTO 1
00630 STOP
00650 REM *** INSTRUCTIONS *****
00651 GOSUB 900
00652 PRINT"SCATCHARD INSTRUCTIONS"
00653 PRINT "***********************"
00670PRINT
00700 PRINT"    THIS PROGRAM WILL CALCULATE VALUES
FOR BOTH THE K.D."
00710 PRINT"AND B. MAX DIRECTLY FROM THE SCINTILLA-
TION COUNTER RESULTS."
00720PRINT
00730 PRINT"  YOU WILL BE ASKED TO ENTER NON-SPECIFIC
BOUND COUNTS"
00740 PRINT" AND TOTAL COUNTS FOR EACH DATA POINT.
AFTER ENT"
00750 PRINT" INDIVIDUAL VALUE, PRESS RETURN."
00760PRINT
00770PRINT"    AT THE END OF EACH SET OF VALUES FOR
TOTALS OR NSBS,"
00780PRINT "ENTER THE VALUE N, FOLLOWED BY RETURN,"
00790PRINT
00800PRINT" INPUT LETTER C TO CONTINUE"
00810 INPUT C$
00820 IF C$<> "C" THEN GOTO 800
00860 GOTO 100
00900REM
00910 FOR Z9=1 TO 23
00920 PRINT
00930 NEXT Z9
00940 RETURN
```

Appendix 7.2 Summary of appropriate statistical tests for analysis of different types of data

Type of data

Types of statistic	Continuous		non-normal untransformable	Ordinal		Categorical
	normal	non-normal transformable		individual scores	frequencies	
Original form of data	normal	non-normal transformable	non-normal untransformable	individual scores	frequencies	
Data used in analysis	raw scores	transformed scores (Fig. 7.6)	ranks	ranks	ranks	frequencies
Compare two groups	unrelated/uncorrelated t-test (= ANOVA)		Mann–Whitney U-test (Table 7.2)			2×2 contingency table and χ^2 (Table 7.9)
Compare three or more groups	analysis of variance (ANOVA); main effects, interactions and contrasts (Tables 7.3 and 7.4)		Kruskal–Wallace test plus Page's test for main effects, interactions and contrasts (Tables 7.6 and 7.7)			$r \times c$ contingency table plus χ^2 and partitions
Two repeated measures	related/correlated t-test (=ANOVA)		Wilcoxon test or sign test			sign test

Three or more repeated measures	ANOVA plus trends and contrasts multivariate analysis of variance (MANOVA)	Friedman test plus Page's test for trends and contrasts (Table 7.8)	$r \times c$ contingency table plus χ^2 and partitions
Repeated measures and group comparisons	ANOVA plus trends and contrasts MANOVA (Fig. 7.7)		
Correlation and linear regression	Pearson correlation and linear regression	Spearman rank order correlation	2×2 contingency table plus χ^2 (Table 7.9)
Non-linear regression	non-linear regression (Fig. 7.8)	Friedman test plus Page's test for trends	—
Covariance	analysis of covariance (ANCOVA) and MANOVA (Table 7.5)		log-linear models (Table 7.10)

Index